D1165112

wearing

vintage

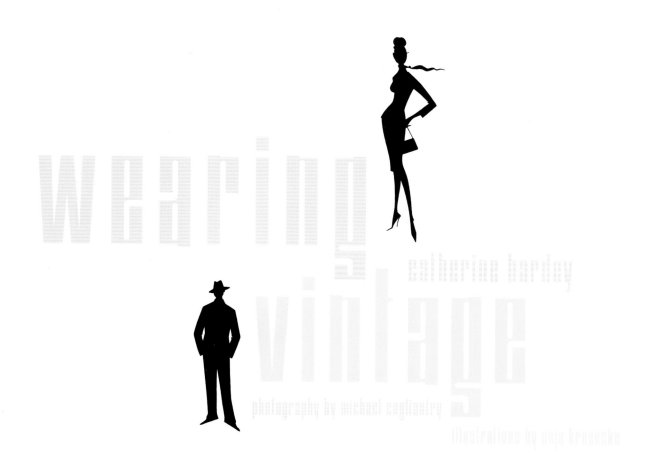

wearing

vintage

catherine harley

photography by michael cogliantry

illustrations by anja kroencke

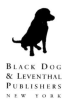

BLACK DOG
& LEVENTHAL
PUBLISHERS
NEW YORK

ISBN 1-57912-233-7

Library of Congress Cataloging-in-Publication Data

Bardey, Catherine, 1963-
   Wearing vintage / by Catherine Bardey; photography by Michael Cogliantry.
       p. cm.
     ISBN 1-57912-233-7
       1. Vintage clothing—United States. 2. Costume—United States—History—20th century.
   I. Title.

   GT615 .B37 2002
   391'.00973—dc21

2001056616

Book design: 27.12 Design Ltd., NYC

Printed in China

Published by
Black Dog & Leventhal Publishers, Inc.
151 West 19th Street
New York, New York 10011

Distributed by
Workman Publishing Company
708 Broadway
New York, New York 10003

g f e d c b a

Author's Acknowledgments

I would like to thank designer Jeniffer Harte, illustrator Anja Kroencke, and photographer Michael Cogliantry, without whose talent, enthusiasm, creativity, and hard work this book would not have been possible.

I am also indebted to the following retailers for their contributions of clothing and accessories, their time, and their expertise. I hope that everyone who picks up this book out of a love of vintage will eventually make their way to the establishments so lovingly and knowledgeably run by them:

Seth Weisser, Lauren Sweder, and Hidei Sagawa of
     What Comes Around Goes Around (NYC)
Renée Soucy and Patti Stoecker of POSH Vintage (Miami)
Suzie and Allan of Allan & Suzie (NYC)
Mike Sportes of Filth Mart (NYC)
Tracy Chappelear of The Family Jewels (NYC)

I would also like to extend heartfelt thanks to the following individuals who opened their closets and their minds for the project: Chad Kincaid, Merideth Harte, Pamela Horn, Amy Harte-Hossfield, Frank DiCrescenzo, Claudia Strauss, Joshua Stone, Jessica Hasselbusch, and Ben Hoffman.

Special thanks to my ever-so-patient editor, Laura Ross, for her unwavering persistence, dedication, and encouragement; my publisher, J. P. Leventhal, for helping me turn my ideas into beautifully realized books and never stinting in the process; and to True Sims, Reeve Chace, Iris Bass, and Lesley Bruynesteyn for helping to put all the pieces together.

Last, but certainly not least, I would like to thank my daughter Isabelle for her constant inspiration and laughter, and my husband John for that too, of course, and for everything else.

contents

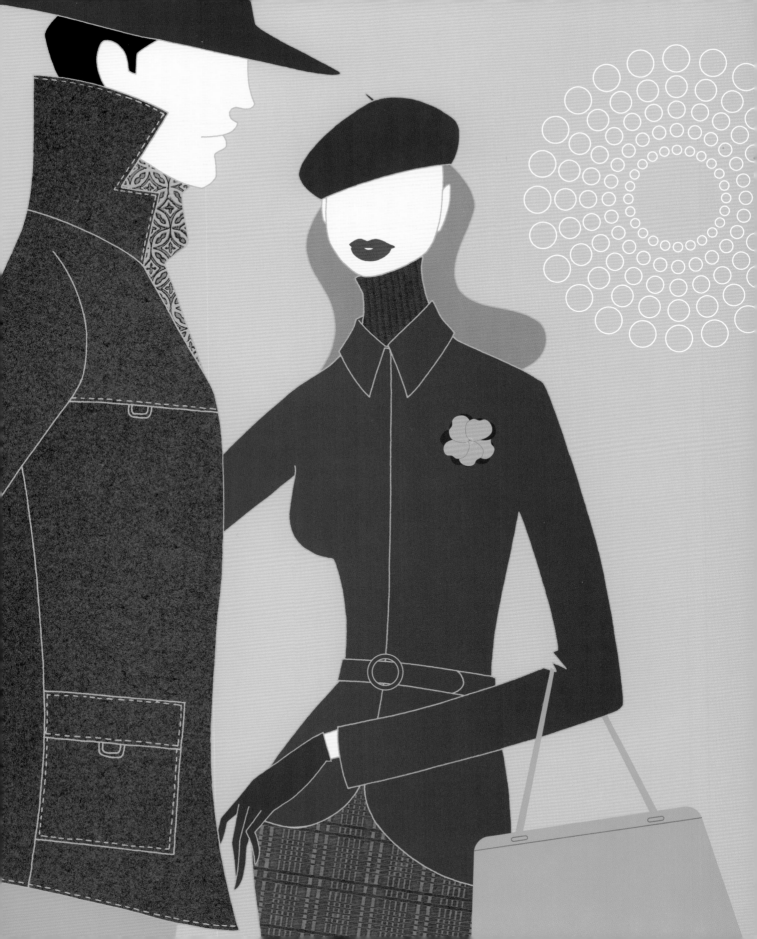

{1}

introduction

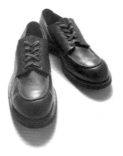

"Eternal nothingness is fine
if you happen to be dressed for it."

—*Woody Allen*

vintage: what & why

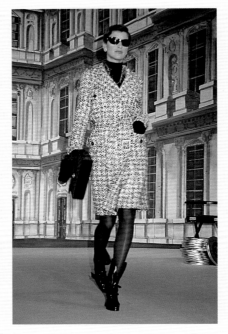

If you've caught a glimpse of recent designer runway shows, flipped through the pages of fashion magazines lately, or watched the Oscars to see what the Hollywood "It" boys and girls are wearing these days, chances are you've noticed that something has changed. At first, you're not quite sure what it is. So you feel for a pulse. You search for a common thread, that recurrent theme woven through the seams of fashion that usually ends up pointing to a specific trend or a designer's imprimatur: structured shoulder pads or tiny waists; lengthening or receding hemlines; puffy skirts or micro jack-ets; military-style coats or Western-inspired dusters; thin ties, baggy trousers or wide lapels.

But this time, it's different. It feels different. It's no longer about one style or one designer's signature; it's about hundreds of styles and thousands of designers. It's about a subtle blend of elegance and ease, a juxta-position of the old with the new, a little tradition mixed in with the avant-garde. And it's about originality and individuali-ty, about flair and fun, painted with broad strokes of creativity and a soupçon of attitude, the result of which not only works, but works well. It's about vintage.

Strut your stuff in vintage duds—in this case, classic Chanel—and show off your irreproachable flair and disarming style. Opposite: Great vintage finds include a 1960s Pioneer Wear fringed buckskin jacket.

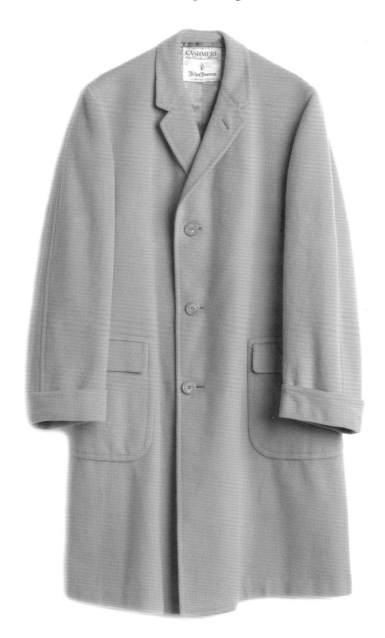

"It's about a subtle blend of elegance and ease, a juxtaposition of the old with the new, a little tradition mixed in with the avant-garde."

{what's vintage?}

"vin.tage (vin'tij)—adj. 1. a) of a good vintage or period; choice [vintage wine] b) representative of the best 2. representative or dating from a period long past [vintage clothes]."[1]

Vintage—a voguish alias for "secondhand," "used" or sometimes "retro"—simply refers to clothes and accessories that were made in the past. Setting time limits for the definition of vintage can be quite challenging, because everyone has a different opinion. When does something fall out of the realm of contemporary and into the vintage arena? Is something ever too old to be considered vintage, and if so, how old is too old? Some insist that vintage refers to clothing and accessories that are fifteen years old or more, or that were made before the

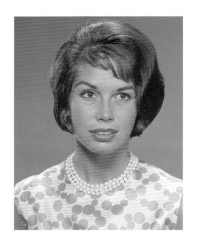

Mary Tyler Moore's day-dress-and-pearls look from the sixties is as fresh as ever.

1990s, and after the 1930s. Others consider vintage to be anything made between the late 1880s and early 1950s. Others still are adamant that it is anything made prior to the 1960s, when wearing old clothes became a fashion statement and not a mark of poverty.

And there are, of course, the purists who argue that vintage is anything that is not on the department store rack today.

Most vintage dealers and collectors agree, however, that vintage refers to the range of clothing and accessories made from the late 1920s (anything prior to that is more akin to "costume" or "antique" than "vintage") through the mid '70s. Anything made after that would simply be too new. Some time needs to pass before the qualities of a piece can properly be determined and assessed; and only with distance can fabrication, style, quality, and durability shine through and be appreciated. As for those of us who gasp at the thought of anything from the '70s being vintage (after all, wasn't that, like, *yesterday*?), for those of us who planned our daily schedules around *Gilligan's Island* or *The Sonny and Cher Comedy*

and the award for best vintage goes to

OSCAR 2001
Julia Roberts, who won Best Actress for her role in Erin Brockovich,
wore a vintage black velvet Valentino couture column gown with a tulle train and white line accents.

Kate Hudson, nominated for Best Supporting Actress for her role in Almost Famous, wore nineteenth-century
diamond feather hair ornaments that were originally brooches owned by Queen Victoria's children.

Russell Crowe, awarded the Best Actor Oscar for his role in Gladiator, wore a knee-length Edwardian-style
Giorgio Armani tuxedo jacket.

Renée Zellweger appeared in a 1950s Jean Desses strapless canary-yellow chiffon gown.
Ashley Judd wore 1920s-inspired diamond jewelry,
which included more than 200 carats of both vintage and contemporary gems.

The flapper vintage look inspired Juliette Binoche's Jean-Paul Gaultier corset dress decked
with 1930s-style beads.

OSCAR 2000
Winona Ryder looked divine in a 1940s Pauline Trigère couture gown lined in cream satin.
Sadie Frost wore a peach silk 1950s dress when she accompanied her husband, Jude Law.

OSCAR 1994
Winona Ryder wore a 1959 fringy, beaded white Edward Sabesta dress. Sabesta was once a big-time
Hollywood eveningwear designer who dressed the likes of Natalie Wood.

OSCAR 1992
Demi Moore looked superb in a 1940s lavender halter dress. She had it altered from a size 12 to a size 4.

OSCAR 1983
To present the Best Supporting Actor award with Christopher Reeve, Susan Sarandon wore a rhinestone-
trimmed vintage dress and a coordinating flapper hairstyle.

Hour, who sucked Sugar Daddies and lost teeth in Now and Laters, and who knew that when the mood ring turned blue, you were in love with your science teacher, the seventies seem like yester-day. The fact is, they ended more than thirty years ago. Indeed, the clothing or acces-sories from that era are considered "vintage." The appeal of vintage has inspired trend-setting divas and super-hunks to sport things they wouldn't have been caught dead wearing ten or twenty years ago, and to give classic pieces a com-pletely different twist. The craze for vintage is directly responsible for resurrecting a great aunt's bias-cut evening gown (the one that's been hiding in the back of her closet forever) or her fur-trimmed sweater (the one that smells like moth balls), a pair of tight, mod '60s pants à la James Bond, graffiti-splattered bell-bottom jeans from high school, or a grandfather's Hamilton watch (the one he received for his retirement more than fifty years ago). In essence, vintage has pulled from musty basements and dusty attics what is now holding court at the front of the closet. Vintage has become so hot that the millenni-um's top fashion designers—from John Galliano, Marc Jacobs, Donna Karan, Ralph Lauren, Miuccia Prada, Calvin Klein, and Tom Ford to Stella McCartney, Narcisco Rodriguez, and Richard Tyler—

why vintage

- *The thrill of the hunt and of the unexpected*
- *The variety of styles and sizes*
- *The quality of fabrics and craftsmanship*
- *Knowing that what you have is authentic or that it's an original*
- *The fun of recreating old looks or reinventing them mixed with modern pieces*
- *The satisfaction of finding a bargain: getting the best for less*

are rummaging through the recesses of time and antiquated trends to find inspiration. In fact, these Gods of Creation are blatantly duplicating styles and cuts from previous eras, using vintage fabrics to make new pieces, or using actual vintage pieces to supplement a look. A case of the "inspiration well" gone dry? Not at all.

So why is fashion, by definition dedicated to all that is new, different, and unexpected, turning to the past for identity? And why are so many of today's fashion icons—from movie stars and models to savvy college students and that hot guy who pours drinks at the local bar—engaging in the hunt for vintage? How do they manage to wear it with such style that it constitutes a whole new look?

Forty years ago, the idea of slipping into someone else's clothing was positively unheard of, bordering on the reprehensible or even pitiful. "Hand-me-downs" were a mark of poverty, scorned like the scarlet "A," an unfortunate stain your mother would have wiped off with a bit of saliva and a handkerchief, given the opportunity. More recently, the image of vintage improved only slightly, epitomized by Cyndi Lauper or a student on a tight budget. But today, the rules have changed drastically. Wearing things from the past no longer incites a raised eyebrow of disapproval or pity, but a nod of approval, maybe even a bit of envy. Nostalgia may have a lot to do with the appeal of vintage today. In an age zooming forward technologically and changing with mind-boggling speed, we find comfort and stability in the familiarity of the past, we revel in

A cornucopia of vintage treasures. Clockwise, from top right: A pair of black satin 1950s Jacques Levine mules; a pair of forty-year-old "Regal" loafers snazzed up with snakeskin; a pair of 1960s vinyl boots—made for walkin'; and a fab fifties leopard print faux-fur coat with rolled collar and cuffs. Opposite: A 1950s Varsity college V-neck by Mitchell's of Hobart.

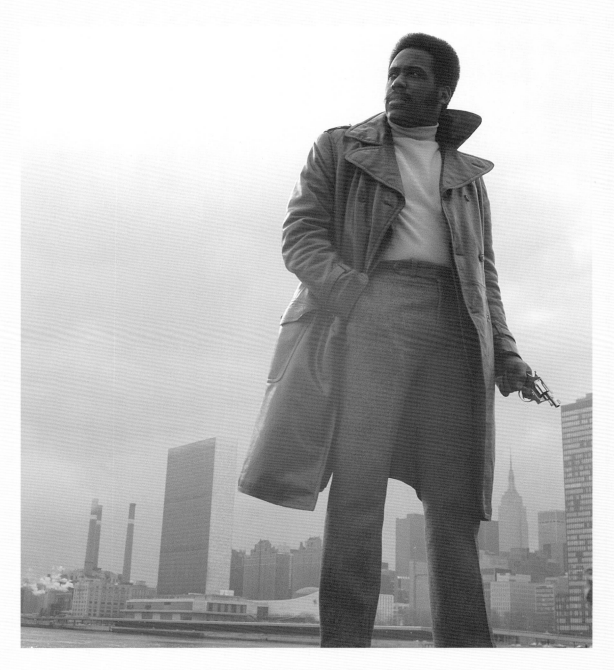

*"Can you dig it?" Richard Roundtree influenced style as Shaft,
the suave detective in the 1971 movie of the same name.*

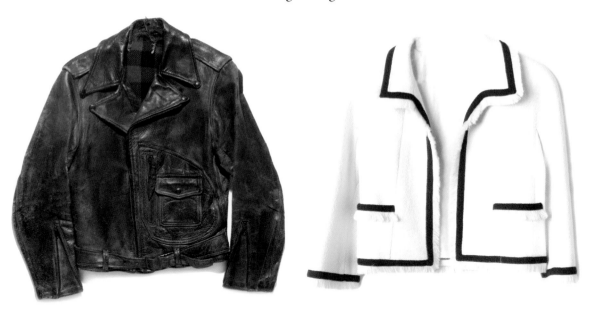

*Biker brass from the forties vs. Chanel chic from the sixties:
you can own it all and then let your mood prevail.*

resurrecting the "good old days" as seen through rose-colored lenses. The return of *Charlie's Angels* and *Shaft*, movie-style, or the success of movies like *Almost Famous* and *Austin Powers*, are obvious manifestations. Steeley Dan is back on the podium, and strains of Simon & Garfunkel's "Homeward Bound" sell Microsoft products on television. In fact, our longing for the past has become so acute that "these days, it's not necessary to evoke the past; you can't move without tripping over it."[2] Perhaps, then, vintage is to fashion what mashed potatoes are to comfort food.

But nostalgia cannot account for why many of today's fashion trendsetters are dressing in vintage, since most are too young to have experienced the "real thing" the first time around. It's highly unlikely that Kate Hudson, David Arquette, Winona Ryder, or Gwyneth Paltrow wear vintage because they are looking for their "lost youth." It's possible, however, that the age-old adage "what goes around, comes around" contributes to the popularity of classic fashion. As we move through history, cycles repeat themselves and familiar styles re-emerge, withstanding the ravages of time and overcoming change while maintaining their grace, style, and dignity. These timeless pieces fit right in, whenever and wherever they resurface: a Chanel suit, a classic trench coat, cashmere twin-sets, Hawaiian print shirts, the Kelly bag, black cocktail dresses, and leather biker jackets.

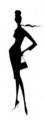

selecting a silhouette: women

HOURGLASS FIGURE, CURVY WITH A SMALL WAIST
Floor-length evening gowns from the 1930s; 1940s dresses and
suits with nipped-in or belted waists; 1950s sheath dresses;
A-line dresses from the 1960s.

LONG, THIN, AND BOYISH
1920s flapper and shift dresses; close-fitting tapered trousers with short tops from the 1950s;
1960s shift dresses and mini skirts; peasant looks and sleek knits of the 1970s.

PEAR-SHAPED WITH HEAVIER HIPS AND BOTTOM
1950s day dresses with low waists; A-line dresses from the 1960s; kaftans from the 1970s.

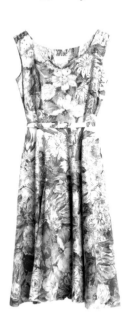 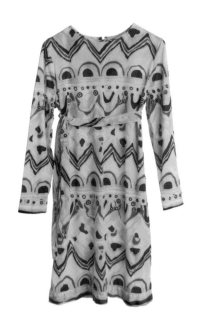 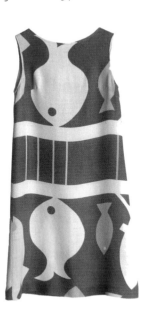

From left to right: A 1950s day dress, perfect for trim waists and toned arms; a high-waisted seventies number that's great for short-waisted figures; and an A-line from the 1960s, flattering nearly every figure.

selecting a silhouette: men

BROAD-SHOULDERED
*Suits from the 1940s with jacket buttons set lower and lapels cut longer to accentuate height.
The look was tall and slim, to be worn with spread collar shirts;
bowling shirts from the 1950s and 1960s.*

SHORT
*One-button suits from the 1960s; avoid three and four-button suits;
"flood" khakis from the 1960s.*

TALL, LEAN, AND THIN
*Natural-shouldered suits from the 1950s with thin lapels;
tight mod suits from the 1960s with tapered pants.*

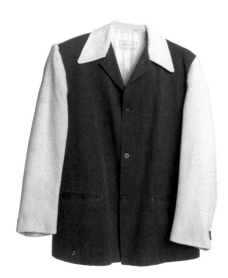
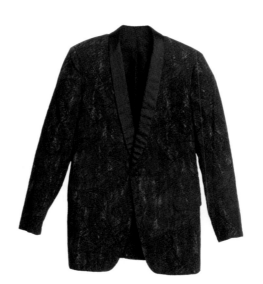
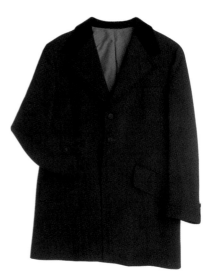

Different strokes for different blokes: Spread-collared, single-breasted, or three-buttoned jackets should be chosen to emphasize the shoulders and be kind to the waistline.

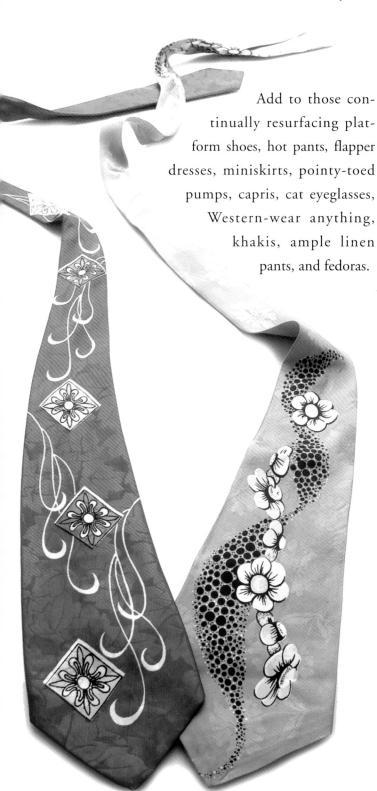

Add to those continually resurfacing platform shoes, hot pants, flapper dresses, miniskirts, pointy-toed pumps, capris, cat eyeglasses, Western-wear anything, khakis, ample linen pants, and fedoras.

Notwithstanding nostalgia and history's cyclical rhythms, fashion aficionados have resurrected clothing from the past for more basic reasons. First and foremost, vintage is about variety of style and fit. Men and women shoppers today feel restricted and bored by the cookie-cutter designs hanging on department store racks and are looking for something unique, something that will set them apart from the crowd. They are tired of mass-market "branding" and don't want to be another walking advertisement for a designer's label—or for The Gap and Banana Republic. They crave one-of-a-kind items and pieces that exude so much quality in fabrication, cut, and fit that their style remains timeless.

While contemporary designers do strive for originality, it's not uncommon for a particular look or a hot new fabric to filter down to the mass market, and after awhile, it all starts to look the same. Retailers, restricted by seasonal constraints and overstock concerns, carry only one season at a time and offer limited styles and sizes. (It should be noted, however, that recently high-end department stores like Bendel's and Barney's have started carrying vintage, so as to offer a little something different and special for their finicky customers. Besides, it's a sure thing for retailers, since vintage items need not ever be marked down.) Vintage is like having one hundred seasons to pick from under the same roof! A single rack might yield a silk chiffon gown from the 1950s, a plaid Pendleton shirt from the 1960s, a bright orange or yellow Courrèges dress from the 1960s, and a no-name dark blue peacoat that looks like something "99" might have worn in *Get Smart*. Digging through a bin, you might unearth a 1940s tie, a silk dressing gown Rudolph Valentino might have worn, a fringed shawl that could pass for art deco, a 1920s man's wool cloak with satin brocade, and sailor pants with back laces and front decorative buttons. And not only is the clothing representative of multiple eras and fashion trends, but it's Men's, Women's, Winter, Spring, Summer, Fall, Eveningwear, Daywear, Loungewear, Outerwear, and Swimwear all at once.

Often, too, the looks promoted by contemporary designers are tailored to fit a narrow range of body types or lifestyles. Some human sizes or shapes just look better in clothes from other eras. Day dresses and men's suits from the thirties, for example, tend to be less form-fitting and more forgiving than their forties equivalents stiffened with boning, complex interlining and all kinds of stitching, thus making them ideal for voluptuous curves or sturdy builds. Long and lean figures with minimal shape practically cry out for the ultra-minis and tapered pants of the sixties, while A-line dresses, which put no emphasis on the breasts, waist or hips, provide a flattering solution for virtually any body type. And the mod, skinny, one-button men's suits with tapered pants from the 1960s can only be carried off by the lean and slick.

Bold silk ties from the 1950s also make great belts for women. Layered or on its own, a retro slip can pose as a slinky little cocktail dress or a swanky nightgown.

vintage must-haves

1920s:
Flapper dresses, silk blouses, beaded purses, beaded shawls, slips, teddies, peignoirs, camisoles, chemises, "cloche" hats, coats with fur collars, mesh evening bags, wool cloaks, Panama hats, high-waisted cotton trousers, leather car coats, mourning coats.

1930s:
Chinese quilted jackets, slim pants, lounging pajamas, sheath dresses, coat and dress sets, sweater twin-sets, bias-cut evening dresses, tap pants, palazzo pants, slips, gloves, piano scarves, mesh bags, four-button jackets with wide lapels, double-breasted suits, tuxedos.

1940s:
Tailored suits, hand-knit tops, swagger coats, full skirts, bed jackets, saddle shoes, trench coats, cashmere sweaters, fur-trimmed hats, bathing suits, Fair Isle sweaters, suspenders, cotton shirts.

1950s:
Classic tweed or jersey Chanel-style skirt suits, day dresses with floral prints, tight-fitting Chinese dresses with matching vests, dresses with matching bolero jackets, A-line dresses, beaded cardigans, fur-trimmed cardigans, capri pants or pedal pushers, cigarette pants, swing coats, wrapped bathing suits, Bakelite and Lucite bags, bamboo-handled bags, minaudière bags, charm bracelets, costume jewelry, stiletto heels, Western-wear, hand-painted ties, Hawaiian shirts, khakis, leather jackets.

1960s:
Shift dresses, miniskirts and dresses, hand-crocheted dresses, skirts and tops, boots and accessories with space-age designs, Lucite accessories, hand-painted T-shirts, jeans, ponchos, Afghan coats, bowling shirts, men's collarless jackets, tartan suits.

1970s:
Dresses with ethnic or exotic prints, pantsuits with exaggerated lapels and flared legs, A-line skirts, maxi skirts, wrap dresses, halter tops, tube tops, palazzo pants, maxi coats, T-shirts, bodysuits, fringed jackets, kaftans, varsity jackets, platform shoes, Frye boot, clutch bags, frilly tuxedo shirts.

Quality of craftsmanship and material is another reason why many people are turning to vintage. "They just don't make things like they used to" might be a familiar cliché, but it couldn't be more appropriate in this case. Before big designers took over the land, and certainly before mass production came into play in the late forties, clothes were often individually designed and entirely fabricated by hand. The care and time that went into manufacturing clothing was monumental. Each seam and hem was individually sewn, often two or three times over; each bead and sequin was individually placed and hand sewn or knit in; buttons were often covered with fabric; linings were specifically cut and tailored to exact measurements; and pleats were hand-pressed to absolute perfection. Tweeds were reinforced by cotton batiste for an ideal drape; simple sheaths were subtly cut and designed to sway with the body; and coat linings were made of heavy silk and a lightweight inner panel for warmth. Fabrics were finer, weaves were tighter, cashmere was more often four-ply than not, and for the most part, materials—especially before the advent of rayon—were natural instead of synthetic. Not only are some of the materials no longer avail-able today, but the time and cost of attending to this level of detail makes it virtually impossible to duplicate the creativity and design of these one-of-a-kind pieces. Simply put, vintage in 2002 is what couture was in the '40s—a means of assuring that what you purchase is a high-quality original product.

People are also shopping for vintage because it's fun, and it gives them room to flex their creative muscles and to develop an individual style. Some compare the whole vintage shopping experience to a treasure hunt: the often frenetic sift through thousands of articles of clothing for that one-of-a-kind piece or key signature item, or the instant adrenaline rush of finding a buried treasure at the bottom of a pile of wrinkled men's shirts. Of course, nothing tops the immense satisfaction you get when someone stops you to ask where you got that fabulous shirt and you reply, "Salvation Army, $4.95!" It's the thrill of the chase and the idea that you never know what you're going to find that turns the vintage shopping experience into a true—some might say addictive—adventure. Others see it as a way to tap into a coursing vein of shared cultural memory and an opportunity to give new life

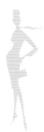

to something that comes from the past. They might relish the thought of buying a little piece of history, too, of acquiring something original, and of knowing that what they now own is authentic, not a latter-day imitation or rip-off. They might also enjoy the idea of purchasing a bit of mystery, especially if the garment has no label.

Shopping and wearing vintage is kind of like being your own designer, because you get to pick and choose and combine items from a variety of eras, creating a new identity through clothes and accessories. You can mix contemporary pieces with relics from the past, and there's never any risk of bumping into someone at a party who is wearing the same outfit. You can dress to suit your mood on any given day, or slip into a different character whenever you feel like it. With vintage, you can add style and versatility to your current wardrobe without spending a fortune (see Chapter 2: "Shopping Tips"), and you can create a one-of-a-kind look for every occasion and every season. You can blend timeless elegance with modern-day ease, juxtapose the old with the new, mix a little tradition with the avant-garde, and have an absolute blast in the process. (And, besides, you'll always have something fabulous to wear when you receive that last-minute invitation to the Oscars.)

Wear a creation such as this exquisite Pauline Trigère chiffon gown from the late sixties and you'll never have to worry about anyone else showing up in the same outfit.

vintage hot labels

1920s:
Jean Patou, Paul Poiret, Coco Chanel, Elsa Schiaparelli.

1930s:
Jean Patou, Coco Chanel, Adrian, Madame Grès, Madeleine Vionnet,
Norman Norell, Mainbocher, Elsa Schiaparelli,
Hattie Carnegie, Whitting & Davis.

1940s:
Christian Dior, Claire McCardell, Whitting & Davis, Joset Walker.

1950s:
Lanvin, Jacques Fath, Victor Stiebel, Gucci, Bonnie Cashin, Mainbocher,
Christian Dior, Duke Kahanamoku, Burberry, Nudie Cohn, Roberta di Camerino,
King Louie, Pauline Trigère, Galanos, Norell (signed Traina-Norell),
Charles James, Nat Nast, Hilton, Cristobal Balenciaga, Claire McCardell,
Elizabeth Hawes, Ferragamo, Coco Chanel, Pierre Balmain.

1960:
Mary Quant, André Courrèges, Hubert de Givenchy, Ossie Clark, Biba,
Louis Féraud, Paco Rabanne, Celia Birtwell, Betsey Johnson, Rudi Gernreich, Pendleton,
Diana Dew, Peter Max prints, Pierre Cardin, Cristobal Balenciaga,
Yves St. Laurent, Emilio Pucci, Oleg Cassini, Kenneth Jay Lane,
Enid Collins, Miriam Haskell, Coach.

1970s:
Ossie Clark, Bill Gibb, Jean Muir, Zandra Rhodes, Giorgio di Sant' Angelo,
René Lacoste, Roy Halston, Ralph Lauren, Elsa Schiaparelli,
Calvin Klein, Steven Burrows, Fiorucci, Missoni, Diane Von Furtsenberg,
Huk-A-Poo, Vivienne Westwood, Norma Kamali.

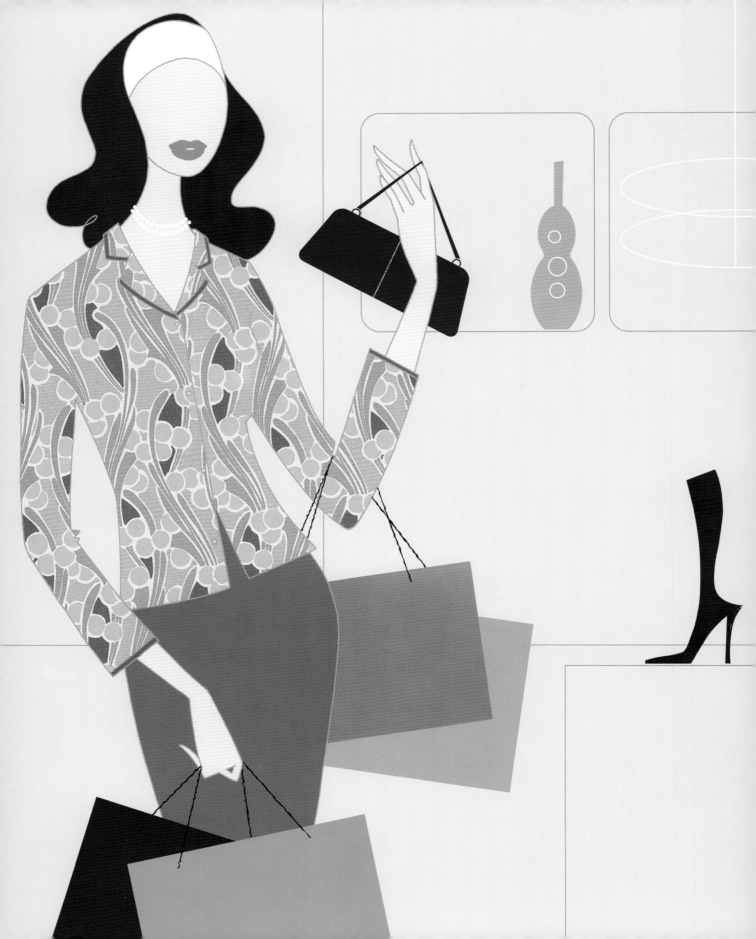

shopping tips

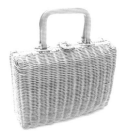

"Fashions fade,
style is eternal."

—*Yves Saint Laurent*

vintage shopping 101

There are a few things you need to know before venturing into the open sea of vintage shopping: where the stuff comes from, where to find it, when to go, what to know before you get there, what to wear (yes, what to wear!), what to do once you're there, what to look for, how to select, and finally, how to make the right decisions, get the most bang for your buck, and acquire fabulous additions for your wardrobe.

First of all, not all "secondhand clothing stores" are the same, and it's important to familiarize yourself with all of them so that you know what to expect. Setting aside yard sales, garage sales, auctions, rummage sales, bazaars, estate sales, flea markets, and your great uncle's closet for a minute, there's a host of names for stores that are in the business of selling used clothing and accessories—"secondhand" shops, "used clothing" stores, thrift stores, resale shops, consignment shops, and vintage shops or boutiques—and they are all different in subtle and not-so-subtle ways. (In fact, if you're using the Yellow Pages as a place to start your shopping journey, look up all of the above-listings. Also check under "Clothing Bought and Sold.") They get their goods from different sources, sell different types of merchandise, price things differently, attract different customers, and have different store policies.

the scoop on stores

• Be prepared to travel: stores that carry the best merchandise are those that haven't really been discovered yet.

• They are often off the beaten track and outside the main shopping areas.

• Explore a variety of shops; each one is unique, just as its merchandise is.

• Visit stores several times a week because sometimes merchandise is restocked on a daily basis.

• Call ahead to find out what store hours are; they are somewhat different from retail store hours.

• Sign up on store mailing lists for customer-only premiums, sale notices, and valuable information that might be sent out in newsletters or flyers.

"A vintage shop can be a feast for style-hungry eyes and a cornucopia for the senses."

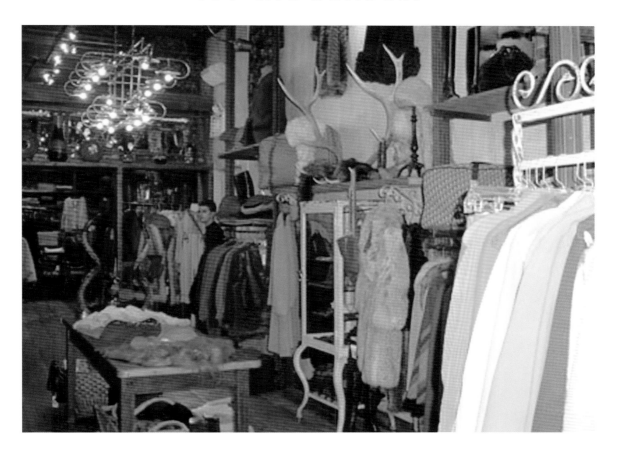

Attention all shoppers: Enter at your own risk! If a glimpse inside What Comes Around Goes Around, a popular New York City vintage treasure trove, doesn't pull you in, check your pulse.

{the inside story}

"Credential bales, rag houses, sorters, consignment stores, thrift shops, and dead stock. Walk the walk and definitely talk the talk."

According to the National Association of Resale and Thrift Shops, based in Michigan, the differences are essentially as follows. Thrift shops or stores are run by not-for-profit organizations and are in the business of selling used goods to raise money to fund charitable causes. These range from the Salvation Army, Children's Hospitals, or Goodwill shops to smaller, volunteer-run thrift shops. Most thrift shops get their merchandise through donations, some operate on a consignment basis, and others do both. Donations are rarely sorted before they are sold. If they are, it's usually by type (men's, women's, children's, skirts, shirts, pants, accessories, etc.) rather than by condition or quality, and sometimes by color (all the red sweaters in one area, the green shirts in another, etc.). As a result, the merchandise you will find in a thrift shop is extremely

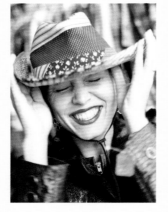

Strike gold or just strike a pose, but always remember to have fun while shopping for vintage.

eclectic and can range from the most glamorous to the most torn, tattered, and stained. Since a thrift shop isn't in the business to make a profit from its sales, the effort put into selling the clothes is generally minimal, and this is often reflected in the store's displays (or lack thereof) or the staff's interaction (or lack thereof) with customers. Defects and damages to particular items are not readily pointed out, so it's very important to thoroughly check the garment before purchasing it. But, because the merchandise is rarely sorted, and vintage-hungry collectors don't want to deal with the hassle of going through mounds of stuff, you can strike gold at thrift shops. And often thrift-shop operators themselves don't know what they have or if a treasure is deeply buried in the recesses of their goods.

Once thrift stores have stocked their racks,

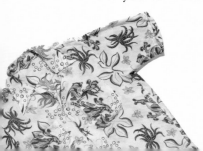

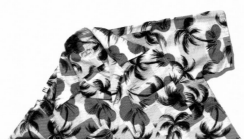

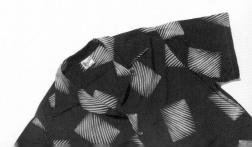

unsorted surplus is baled up into large bags called "credential bales," and are sold by the pound to "rag houses" or "rag merchants." Rag houses or merchants are made up of a network of recyclers, rag makers, wholesalers, and exporters of used clothing. These houses and merchants specifically hire people ("sorters") to sort through credential bales for the purpose of separating the least desirable items (i.e., those that are severely damaged or stained) from the rest. These undesirable items are then broken down into pulp. They are sold by the pound to businesses that reprocess the pulp into fibers, which in turn get restructured into goods (did you ever wonder where your stringy mop head or Handy Wipes come from?). It's basic recycling at its best.

Once the clothing has gone through the first sorting process and the undesirables have been removed, the process is repeated, this time to separate the clothing by type, by season, and by quality. During this second process, trained and seasoned sorters pick through, pick out, and set aside whatever pieces they think might be of interest to secondhand or vintage dealers and collectors. After secondhand or vintage dealers and collectors have made their selections and pur-

chased them, surplus items are bound into 100-pound bales and auctioned off, mostly to exporters of used clothing. The bales are then shipped overseas to developing countries, where importers sell them to wholesalers. These wholesalers, in turn, sell to vendors in local markets and local shops. Madagascar, for example, imported more than nine million pounds of used clothing in 1998, over 650,000 pounds of it from the United States alone.

Lately, though, rag houses and their sorters have become extremely savvy about the value of certain pieces to dealers of vintage clothing or to individual collectors, especially from the European or Japanese markets. In the past, sorters would pull out clothing that was of obvious value, such as a fur coat or a contemporary designer piece, which they knew vintage dealers or collectors would pay more

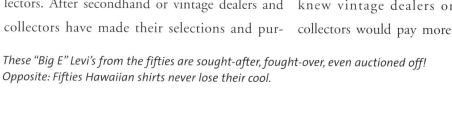

These "Big E" Levi's from the fifties are sought-after, fought-over, even auctioned off! Opposite: Fifties Hawaiian shirts never lose their cool.

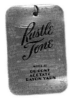

for than a bulk buyer or used-clothing exporter. Recently, sorters have sharpened their skills and have developed a keen eye for setting aside items that might be of value to different types of customers. They then encourage the customers to bid against one another. Vintage Levi's or Nike and Adidas sneakers from a particular year, for example, are very hot items on the Japanese market. Rag houses will therefore give their Japanese clients first bids on the jeans and sneakers because they know the Japanese are likely to pay premium prices. A pair of 1970s Levi's can fetch as much as one thousand dollars, if not more.

Because the market for purchasing used clothing has become so competitive among international buyers and private collectors who swoop down on rag houses to get to the best merchandise first, many vintage clothing stores have been left with what some consider to be less desirable goods, and are opting for different merchandising tactics to sell what they have. Some stores are specializing in clothes with a certain style or from a specific era; some are selling both

"Deadstock" refers to never-worn items with original store tags, like this pair of fifties Rustle Tone swim trunks, and the forties silk socks below.

wholesale to other stores and retail to individuals; others are incorporating new items into their stock, while others still have expanded with costume rentals.

In addition to buying their clothing directly from rag houses, vintage stores buy their merchandise from wholesalers (stores that have gone out of business or stores that have excess stock from seasons past) and from individuals or estates.

It is not out of the ordinary for people with extensive and expensive wardrobes to purge their closets every year. A vintage dealer will simply go to the person's house and buy whatever he or she wants from the assortment offered. The dealer ends up with a fine selection of pieces, many of which boast designer labels from recent seasons, and the original owner ends up with more closet space and extra cash with which to fill it. Consequently, the merchandise in vintage stores is in better condition, or at least in a more predictable condition, than the garments sold in thrift shops. Some items still have their original sales tag on them. These never-worn pieces are referred to as "deadstock."

A consignment shop or store gets its merchandise from individuals or wholesalers who get a percentage of the sale when the item is sold. Consignment shops across the country have different store policies, but most pay the owners 40 percent to 60 percent of the selling price and will display an item for sale for up to sixty or ninety days before returning it to the original owner. Resale shops are similar to consignment shops but they get their merchandise exclusively from individuals, not from wholesalers. Many consignment and resale shops follow an unwritten rule to keep their merchandise flowing in and out of the store on a regular and steady basis, and to keep their racks from getting stale. After an item has been displayed (and remains unsold) for two months, the store will usually knock 20 percent off the marked price. After three months, the store will knock 40 percent off the original price. After four months, 50 percent off; and after six months, the item will go back to the original owner. Therefore, if you happen to spot something you like but don't want to spend what it says on the price tag, sometimes it's worth waiting it out and hoping that no one else will buy

hunting tools

• *Cash.*

• *A measuring tape.*

• *A large, foldable, and light plastic bag in which to carry your goodies. You can stick it in your coat or jacket pocket along with the measuring tape until you need to use them. Avoid carrying a purse or a bulky wallet that might bog you down or that you have to keep an eye on.*

• *Sharp eyes and a good mood.*

• *Educate yourself: learn the big-name designers, the signature styles. If you're going to splurge on an expensive piece, do so at a reputable shop or auction.*

• *Learn about fabrics. The more you know about fabrics, and how to take care of them, the better.*

• *Understand the long-term care required. Some fabrics are too fragile to be washed or cleaned.*

the item so that you can get it at a discounted price two or three months down the line.

Once you've figured out your destination, it's time to get geared up for the hunt. Most stores that sell vintage or secondhand clothing do not have the best changing room facilities for trying something on. If they do have dressing rooms at all, there's usually just one, most likely cramped, with a long line to get into it. And if you're at a flea market, a yard, or garage sale, forget it. Therefore, it's important to dress in such a way that slipping into and out of things is not a hassle. The ideal "hunting" out-fit for women is a body suit or leotard, a wide skirt, and comfortable shoes that can easily come off (clogs, flip-flops, slide-on flats) so as not to have to tie up shoelaces a million times. You can discreetly pull a sweater or T-shirt over the bodysuit to check out the fit; casually slip into a shirt or try on a bathing suit top; gracefully pull a gown

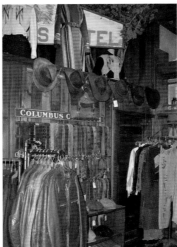

Always survey the territory before going in for the kill. Shops can be jammed with goodies, and it takes a moment to get oriented.

over your head and then remove the skirt underneath for the full effect; slide on a pair of shorts, pants, or a skirt with ease underneath the wide skirt, and all of this while surrounded by a hoard of shoppers and clothing racks. Men should wear fitted T-shirts, boxers or swimming trunks, com-

fortable pants and shoes that come off with ease. While flashing your boxers to try on a pair of pants is not encouraged, it can be done quickly and discreetly behind a curtain or a rack. It also makes sense to know your exact measurements beforehand and to take a measuring tape with you so that in the worst-case scenario where you can't try something on, you can measure the item to see if it might fit.

Once you are completely outfitted, it's time to hit the bank for some cash. Simply put, you have more bargaining power with cash than with any-thing else, and absolutely, posi-tively no transaction should ever be made without bargain-ing first. With the exception of thrift shop volunteers who are trying to raise money for chari-table causes, shop owners, flea market sellers, and garage sale operators expect to bargain. Carry small denominations to make the transactions easier, and leave checks and credit cards at home.

So now you're dressed to kill, you have a bunch of cash burning a hole in your pocket, and you're

mind frame

• *Look at the whole experience like a treasure hunt.*

• *Take it slow: if you're just getting into the idea of wearing vintage, start with an accessory—like a purse or a tie—and work your way up to bigger pieces once you have gotten the feel for it. Shop with an open mind; if you're looking for a specific item, chances are you'll get frustrated trying to find it.*

• *Know the retail prices of items you are shopping for to appreciate how much money you are saving.*

• *Follow your taste: don't buy something just because it's trendy. It's bound to end up in the back of the closet.*

• *Talk to the staff, especially in vintage shops. They're usually in the business because they're passionate about clothes. Don't hesitate to ask questions about the garment's history, its fabrication, its style, or suggestions on how and what to wear it with.*

• *If you see something you like but are hesitant about buying it, don't expect to find it the next day because someone else might have grabbed it. Sometimes it actually pays to be impulsive.*

• *Examine garments closely (see more on page 36, "Giving It The Once Over").*

• *If you're not sure about one particular item, err on the side of buying. If it turns out you made a mistake, you can always sell it back or exchange it.*

• *If you absolutely adore a piece but it's too big, you can always have it tailored later. If a piece is too small, check the generosity of seams and hems for possible altering.*

• *With flea markets, garage sales, or yard sales, it's better to go early in the morning to get the best selection and to get there before collectors and professional "pickers" have had a chance to go through everything. However, prices are often lower at the end of the day because sellers are trying to get rid of their merchandise.*

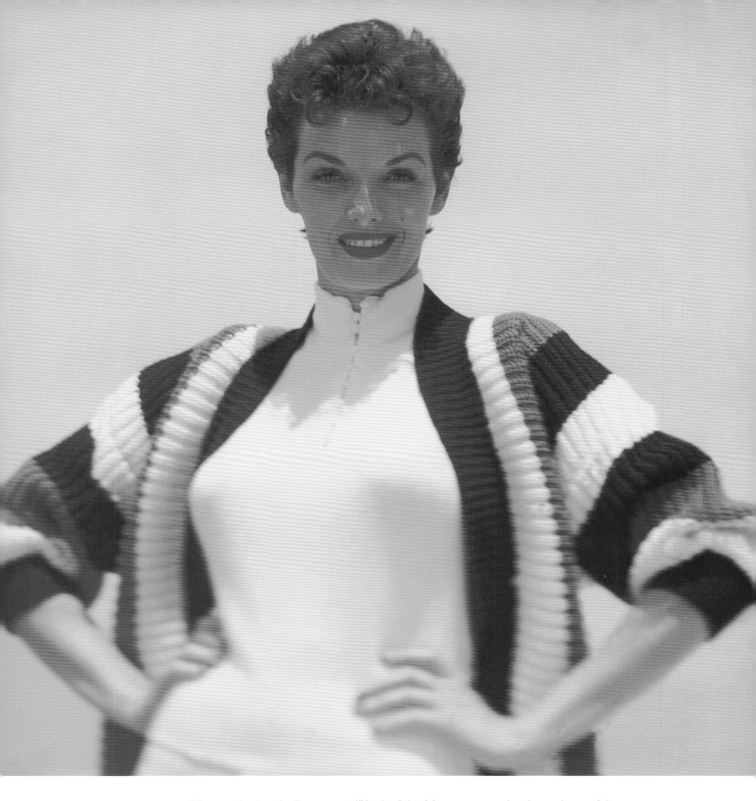

Jane Russell here embodies the "sweater girl" look of the fifties. Her casual style exudes confidence.

famous figures in timeless treasures

PEARLS
Cleopatra, Coco Chanel, Diana Vreeland, Jacqueline Kennedy Onassis, Barbara Bush.

PEA COATS
Frank Sinatra and Gene Kelly in On The Town, *Marlon Brando in* On the Waterfront, *Richard Gere in* The Jackal.

THE LITTLE BLACK DRESS
Audrey Hepburn in Breakfast at Tiffany's, *Marilyn Monroe, Grace Kelly, Jean Simmons, Ali McGraw.*

KHAKIS
James Dean, F. Scott Fitzgerald, Ernest Hemingway, Charles Lindbergh, John F. Kennedy, Jimmy Carter, Katharine Hepburn, Glenn Close.

LEATHER JACKETS
Marlon Brando in The Wild One, *James Dean, Steve McQueen, Elvis Presley.*

SWEATERS
Lana Turner, Jane Russell, Rita Hayworth.

TRENCH COATS
Humphrey Bogart in Casablanca, *Gary Cooper in* Today We Live, *Meryl Streep in* Kramer vs. Kramer, *Katharine Hepburn, Marlene Dietrich, George C. Scott in* Patton, *Michael Douglas in* Wall Street.

ready for the attack. But it's all about the approach. The first thing you need to do when you walk into a vintage clothing store or a secondhand shop is to assess the territory and determine how it's laid out. Most stores organize things by gender (men's and women's) and then by category (skirts, pants, T-shirts, sweaters, coats, jackets, etc.), and sometimes by color and fabric (red shirts, blue skirts, striped pants, leather jackets). Clothing is not often separated according to size because many items don't have size tags on them, and a size 6 in the 1950s has nothing to do with a size 6 today. Always remember to look for the mate to a skirt or a pair of pants in the jacket category (and vice versa), as it might actually be part of a suit that was separated by mistake.

Once you have figured out what's what and where's what, it's time to look at things more closely. As you sift through racks of clothes or overflowing bins of disorganized stuff, there are really three things you should keep in mind: style, quality, and craftsmanship.

Above and beyond everything else, style is primary. If something doesn't have style, it doesn't matter how good the quality of the fabric or craftsmanship is, you just won't wear it. (On the

giving it the once over

- Hold the garment up against the light to check for moth holes and small tears.

- Look on the backside of brocades, bead work, sequin, and stitch work to check the craftsmanship. If it's hand sewn, the garment has more value. Check for lose beads or sequins, and for the extent of repair, if any.

- Check buttons. Look for real brass, pearl, shell, horn, or fabric-covered ones. Check buttonholes, examine linings, and turn the garment inside out to inspect the quality of tailoring.

- Run your fingers down the sides to check for swaying seams.

- Smell the garment: most odors come out with a good cleaning, but body odors and the smell of mothballs tend to linger.

- Shake the garment to assess the quality of the fabric.

- Cast a critical eye on hems, wear on elbows and sleeves, and on overall construction.

- If the garment is stained, keep in mind the cost of having it dry-cleaned (for cleaning tips, see Chapter 9)

- Stay away from pieces that already have lots of repairs. Repairs undermine the value of the piece and indicate that the piece may be too fragile to last.

- Squeeze the garment to discover lumpy linings.

- Check zippers: sometimes they are rotted out or coming out of the seams. Replacing a zipper could be tough when it's an integral part of the garment or when it's a specialty zipper. Courrèges dresses, for example, were made with big white zippers that are hard to find today. The same goes for Gucci buckles.

- With any knits, make sure there hasn't been shrinkage as a result of previous cleanings, thus distorting the shape of the garment.

- Check for tags that are marked "As Is," a dead giveaway that there is a defect in the item.

- Check for stains and tears. Avoid garments that have perspiration stains; these are virtually impossible to get rid of.

- Look at the label itself: if the label is sewn on with thread that looks different from the one used to make the garment, question the authenticity of the piece or of the label, which might have been added at a later date.

- Labels that are woven, not printed, and are sewn down on all four corners instead of just two sides are characteristics of good workmanship and quality.

- Yellowing labels indicate age (which is good), as do labels made from fabric instead of nylon.

- Disregard sizes: a size 6 in 1965 has nothing to do with a size 6 today, and garments can be missized.

other hand, if the piece is made of luscious fabric or has extraordinary trimmings—beautiful covered buttons, fur collar and cuffs, applied lace, sequins, tassels, rhinestone appliqués or elegant beading, for example—but its style is beyond horrendous, and if you happen to be in an enterprising mood, chop up the item and turn it into a pillowcase or scarf, incorporate the trimming into another vintage piece, or jazz up a contemporary one.) Personal style, of course, is a matter of taste and preference. But there are a number of pieces for men and women that are so classic in fabrication, cut, and appeal that they go beyond the realm of personal taste and fall into a timeless and universal style category of their own. They have outlived influences and fads, superceded trends and fash-

ion statements, and have always come out on top. They are dependable, predictable, versatile, and always welcoming of a new twist through accessorizing. Such pieces include the quintessential black dress, the leather biker jacket, a pair of worn-in jeans, a crisp white shirt, a strand of pearls, a trench coat, a knitted skirt suit (Chanel style), turtlenecks, comfy khakis, sweater sets, gray flannel pants, argyle sweaters, pea coats, and button-down Oxford shirts. Obviously, the more authentic the better. If you do happen to come across a Burberry trench coat from the 1940s or a Chanel suit from the 1950s, then you've hit the jackpot, not only because of its monetary value but because of its authenticity. It's kind of like having access to the original Coca-Cola recipe or cruising in a 1957 Chevy. Over the years, many designers and brand names have come up with their own versions of some of these pieces, and

Classic cuts, distinctive style, and timeless elegance are what make key vintage pieces stand out, as in this sampling of treasures from the 1950s: A Catalina men's cardigan in alpaca; a faux leopard handbag; and a pair of colorful stiletto pumps.

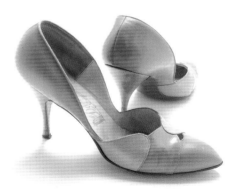

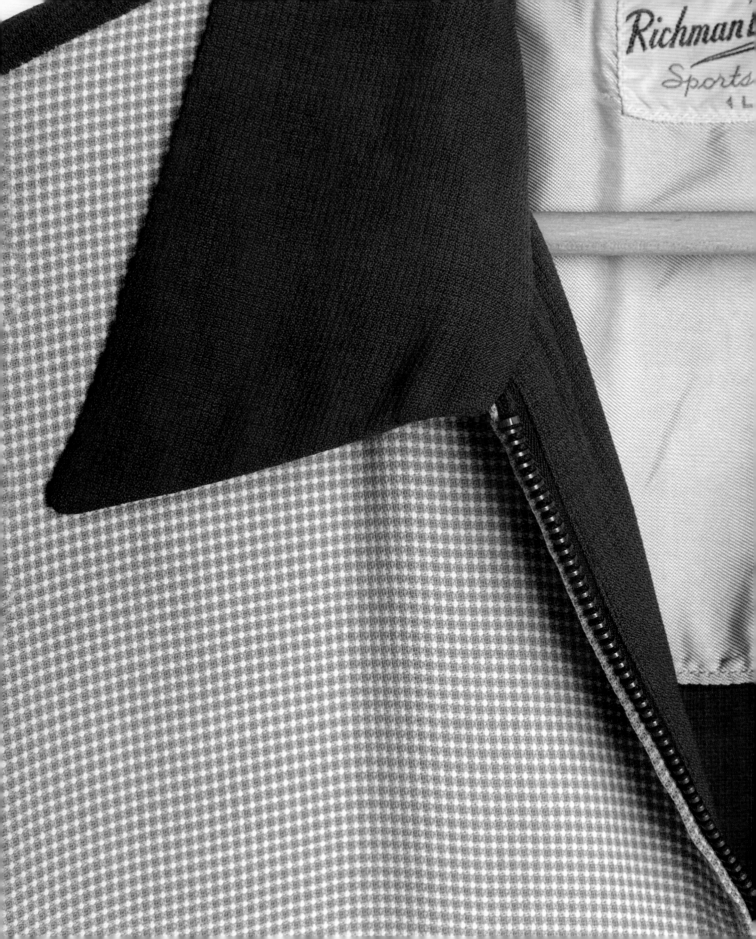

have even found ways of "aging" them to give them more of an authentic feel (e.g. distressed leather, "whiskered" or acid-washed jeans). Stick to pieces that are straightforward in style and as close to the original as possible. And of course, if you are familiar with some of the authentic designers and can recognize labels, you're more likely to end up with a true key signature item.

In addition to style, look for quality of fabric and craftsmanship. It's no secret that clothing made prior to the advent of mass marketing in the 1940s and 1950s is of better quality than clothing made today. Garments were for the most handmade and hand-knitted, seams sewn over two or three times, tucked in at the edges and clean-finished, crafted with intricate boning and interlinings, and trimmings were hand sewn. Worsted wools contained longer, tight-spun fibers, sumptuous silks and rich brocades were heavier and more durable; cashmere was often four-ply. Some fabric experts even swear that rayon made prior to the 1950s, before the original "rayon recipe" was destroyed in a factory fire, was softer, more flowing, and lighter on the skin than rayon made today.

The quality of craftsmanship and attention to detail are equally reflected in vintage accessories: hand-poured glass was used to create costume jewelry; hats were decorated with feathers, beads, pearls, flowers, and sequins; handbags were ornate with wickerwork, chain mail, gold thread, and plastic fruit; ties were handpainted (some even by Salvador Dali); shirt buttons were carved out of coconut shells; and brocade waistcoats were taffeta-lined.

Fabric quality, attention to detail, and superior craftsmanship are the three trademarks of a true vintage find, and all are in evidence in this 1940s gabardine day dress and the Richman Brothers two-tone gabardine men's jacket from the fifties, opposite.

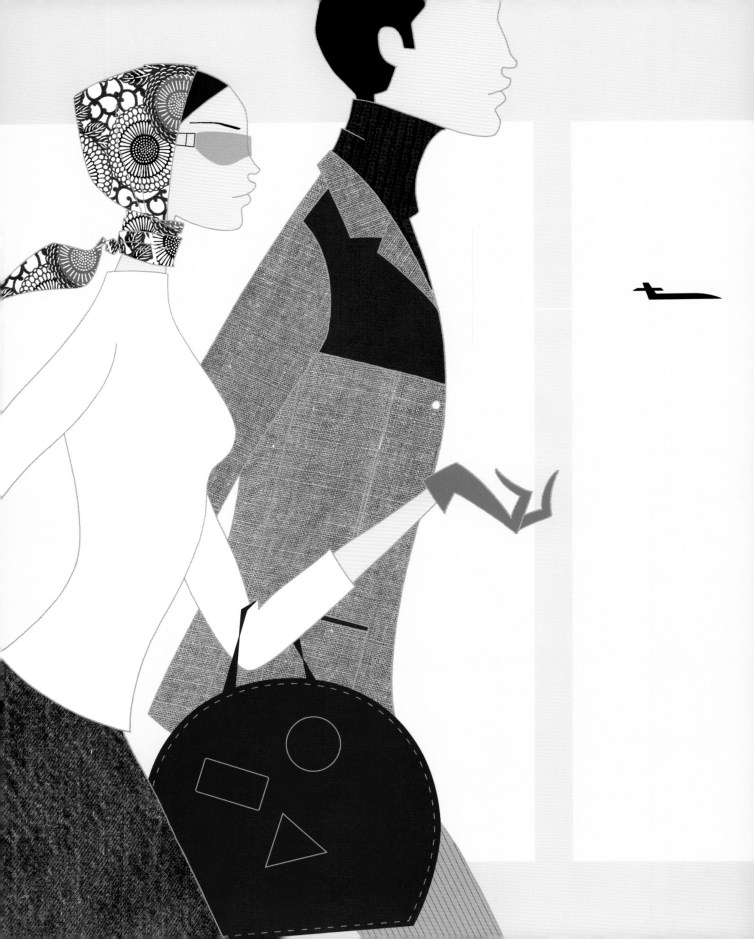

{3}

daywear

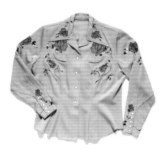

"A woman's dress should be like a barbed-wire fence:
serving its purpose without obstructing the view."

—*Sophia Loren*

daily delights

Whether you're on the prowl for that raspberry sorbet cardigan with glass-beaded embroidery, a pair of Fred Astaire-trademark gray flannel trousers, a palm-tree design Hawaiian shirt à la Burt Lancaster in *Here to Eternity*, or almost anything with fringe, fringe, and more fringe, vintage daywear commands a jurisdiction of its own.

Here, we have carefully selected—among the plethora of poodle-skirted and pinstriped possibilities—a handful of essential daywear items that have proven to be absolute must-haves among vintage

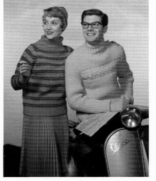

Double the fun—and do it in style—with his-and-hers vintage turtlenecks.

clothing aficionados, keeping in mind the availability of what's out there and how much it costs. For the most part, what makes these particular items stand out is their classic lines, elegance, and superior craftsmanship, as well as their ability to merge beautifully into any modern wardrobe without crying out "Hey,

look at me, I'm sooooooo vintage!" Fun, versatile, and replete with character, they transcend seasons and time, while retaining the function and practicality of everyday wear.

And if you've got a keen eye and savvy approach, your wallet won't be much worse for the wear. A simple A-line dress or fifties' style pedal-pushers and a crisp white Egyptian cotton shirt, for example, can virtually slide into today's world undaunted and unscathed, with a freshness and style that contemporary designers can only dream of replicating. Soft, sturdy khakis paired with a comfortable King Louie bowling shirt or an original flannel Pendleton provide the authenticity and flair lacking in so much of the generic clothing available off the rack. And, yes, there's definitely something to be said for the to-die-for '60s Chanel suit with sewn-in chain for structure and fit.

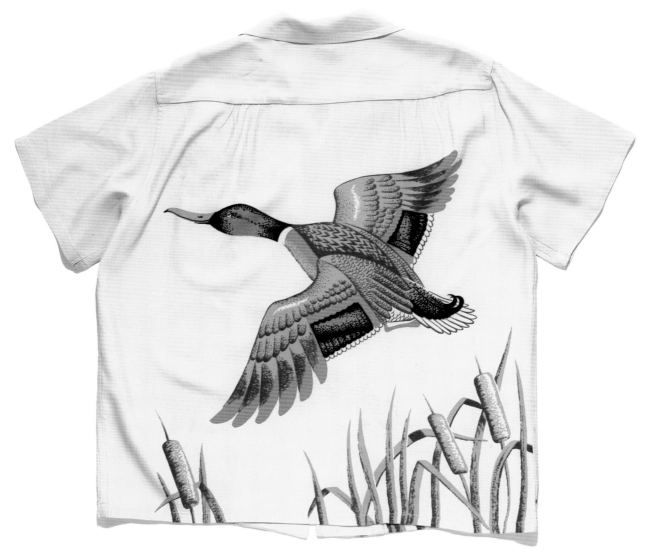

A 1950s "Catalina Hawaiian" men's gabardine shirt, complete with printed mallard.

"The men's vintage market is booming, in large part because there's so much more available now than ever before."

{women's daywear}

"You never know what treasures lurk in the recesses of your great uncle's closet, or at the bottom of the used T-shirt bin at the local flea market."

Ladies, you're in luck. There's definitely more vintage out there for women than there is for men. Maybe it just *seems* that way because women's fashions have always been more diverse than men's—more styles, more versatility, more variations, and certainly much more in the limelight. Or maybe, as one collector joked, it's just that women take better care of their clothes than men do, so they last longer. Or that men just have smaller closets. Either way, there's oodles of women's clothes out there to have fun with, incorporate into your day or evening wardrobe, customize a little for personal flair and style, or just play Greta Garbo or Audrey Hepburn in. And the best part is that just when you *think* you've finished combing through the very last rack, just when it seems that there's no more plucking and poking to be done...there's more! There's a whole world of men's clothing out there just yearning to be revamped and feminized (sorry, guys)! Forget borrowing your boyfriend's oversized V-neck (although definitely a keeper) and worn-in togs when you can actually *have* your very own to play with! There are pinstriped pants just aching to be cinched and belted, large cotton shirts with rolled-up sleeves that look great when knotted at the waist and worn over a pencil-slim skirt, pea coats that do wonders with capris or jeans, chunky watches that flatter smaller wrists, large cardigans that when belted are better than any jacket out there, and ties that are more fun around the waist than on some guy's neck. (Women, get the picture? Make sure you check out the men's sections in this book!) And when you've exhausted the very last of *that* pile, it's always worth taking a peak at children's stuff. A short-sleeved checkered shirt for a size 12 boy is the perfect beach attire over a tiny white T, a pair of white shorts, or cut-offs. And a pleated high-school uniform skirt with a turtleneck, opaque tights, and boots provides just the right punch when packed with a bit of humor and charm.

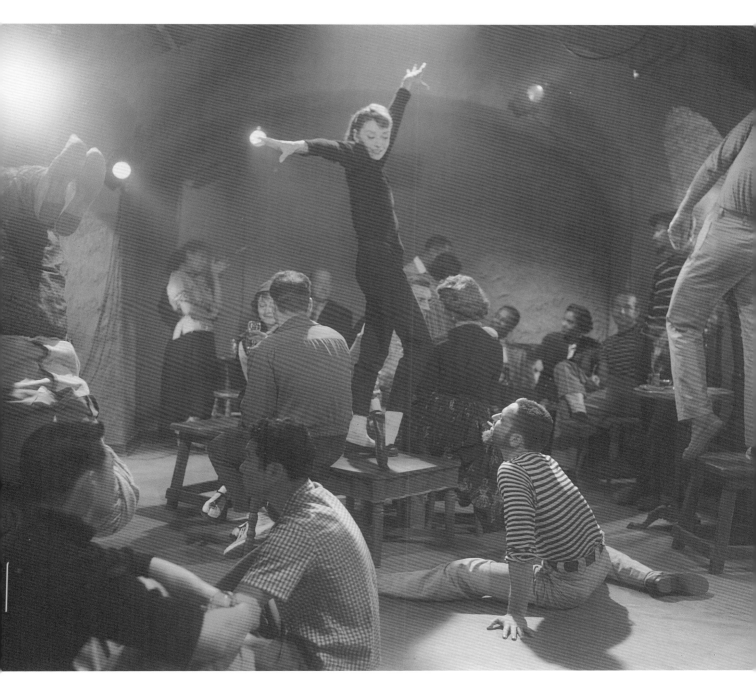

Audrey Hepburn makes a fetching on-screen beatnik in Paris, in cool capris and ballet slippers (Funny Face, 1957).
Opposite: A 1950s white cotton blouse with lace trim and pearl buttons; a late 1950s hand-woven kilt from
Scotland, made by Moffat; and a pair of 1920s black leather shoes with silver buckles.

{cardigans & sweaters}

Indispensable, versatile, and truly irresistible. No wardrobe is complete without a scrumptious vintage cardigan—beaded, embroidered, or in a fabulous pastel—and a fluffy twin set, preferably cashmere, to throw over a little sleeveless dress, to top off a basic skirt, pair up with the perfect slim pant, or dress up with pearls and a brooch.

Sweaters and cardigans were considered "practical" garments in the twenties, when their easy-on, easy-off design proved a simple and unencumbering way of warding off autumn and winter chills. But in the forties and fifties, they took on a completely different spin when Hollywood launched these little staples into the world of glitz and glamour, and transformed them into true fashion necessities. Lana Turner, the cheerleader-turned-actress and curvaceous sex symbol of World War II, is rumored to have been "discovered" while sipping a Coke at a soda fountain and wearing a sweater set. Pretty soon, silver screen images of the Hollywood siren became synonymous with

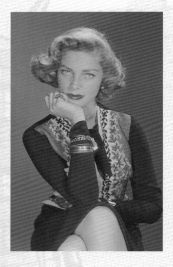

shape-revealing sweaters, earning her the nickname "the original Sweater Girl." Mere footsteps behind Turner, Jane Russell and Rita Hayworth wowed in their knit numbers, and the term "Sweater Girl" was applied to any Hollywood beauty who looked good wrapped in clingy cashmere.

Vintage cardigans, twin-sets, and sweaters are quickly spotted in flea market bins and snatched from the racks, so always be on the lookout for one of these priceless jewels. What makes them so popular, and a favorite with first time vintage shoppers and seasoned "pickers" alike is that they're easy to try on, need little repair and no tailoring, and their impact is undeniable. Most of the cardigans and pull-overs you'll come across are from the forties, fifties, and early sixties, and range anywhere from $10 or $15 to $300 and up, depending on their make, quality, detailing, and condition. Their styles range from simple, draping cuts and elaborately beaded patterns to form-fitting fur-trimmed knits (real or fake) with intricate clasps, glass buttons, and shoulder pads.

sweater matters

Intricate beading, embroidery, fur and trim: If the beading or embroidery is in trouble, make sure it's not beyond repair. If the body is in good shape but some of the buttons are missing, try replacing them with glass or rhinestone buttons from your local trimmings shop. You can always breathe new life into an ordinary but good-quality sweater just by changing the buttons. If, on the other hand, the body is in sad shape but the trim is beautiful and salvageable, sew it onto another sweater for vintage flair.

Moth and insect damage: Hold the garment up to the light to inspect it. If it has small holes, chances are the moths got to the sweater before you did. In addition to creating holes, moths and other insects gnaw on knits, weakening and disintegrating the fiber in ways that are not always visible to the naked eye. If your garment has survived this long without falling prey to vermin, make sure to throw in a few mothballs before storing it.

Shrinkage: Sometimes sweaters have been improperly cared for (e.g., machine-washed instead of hand-washed), thus causing shrinkage in the arms, waistband, and body. Make sure the sweater has retained its original shape. And remember, the best way to store your sweaters is to fold them. Hanging them, especially on wire hangers, is definitely hazardous to their health. It stretches them out and introduces funny looking shoulder bulges.

Many of them were made from 100 percent natural fibers like cashmere (usually two-ply and sometimes three) or lamb's wool blends, and were knitted in Hong Kong or India, as their labels indicate. Face it, you just can't get that kind of quality today without taking out a small loan.

Prior to the introduction of synthetic fibers in the late forties and very early fifties, and prior to the development of new mass-production manufacturing techniques, sweaters were for the most part hand knit and decorated with embroidery or beadwork (beads were made of glass back then). They were often boxy in shape or cropped bolero-style, which makes them ideal for any of today's silhouettes, and were sometimes lined with satin or silk to counteract the weight of the beading and to help maintain the garment's shape. Daytime cardigans were simple and came in solid colors and floral patterns, enhanced with a little

A fifties cream wool cardigan with an intricately stitched floral motif.
Opposite: A silently seductive Lauren Bacall sports a black and gold cardigan (1953).

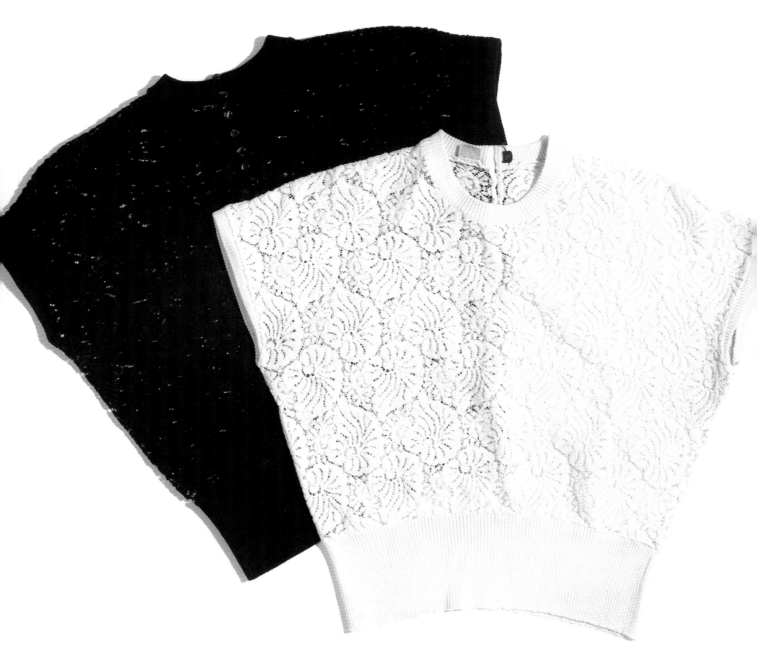

*One of these 1950s sleeveless sweaters with shell motifs and
ribbed hems might pair beautifully with a simple straight skirt or narrow pants.*

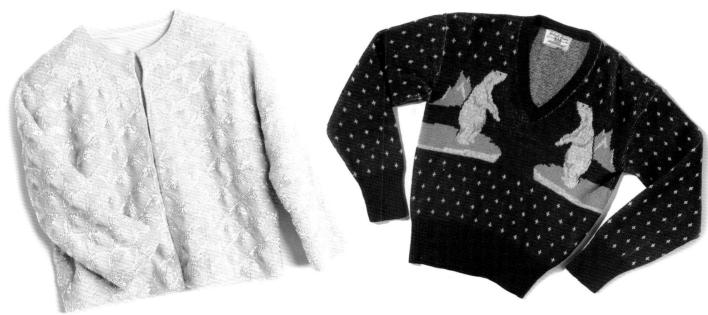

A fully-lined pink cardigan with sequins, circa 1960;
a fifties V-neck pullover with twin polar bears.

piping. They were usually sold with a sleeveless shell to be worn underneath. Mainbocher, who, among other things, designed uniforms for the Women's Marine Corps and for the American Red Cross, was responsible for bringing daytime cardigans into the nightlife arena by adding all sorts of beadwork and intricate sequins. Helen Bond Carruthers, who was famous for making some of the most beautiful cardigans of the 1950s, decorated hers with tiny pearl buttons, rhinestones, embroidery, appliqués, lace, and sequins. If you find a sweater that is not lined, check out the reverse side of the beadwork and you'll be amazed by the intricate stitching: each tiny bead or pearl was actually hand sewn on, and each sequin was knitted right into the sweater. Cardigans from the fifties were originally considered eveningwear, but do wonders today with a pair of jeans, a T-shirt and flats, or over a slim skirt and heels.

When synthetic fibers such as acrylic were introduced, sweaters became more durable and easier to care for (many of them were now machine washable). They retained their shape better, which enabled manufacturers to get more creative with style and cut. Patterned, fancy knitwear, with the design actually incorporated into the knitting as opposed to sewn onto it, was an instant hit with the young college crowd of the fifties and sixties.

{pants}

If you've got the body type to pull it off or you're a clone of Laura Petrie from *The Dick Van Dyke Show*, the cigarette pant—cropped to the ankle and slightly slit on the side—is a sure hit. It's the perfect blend of comfort and style. It can be worn as part of a suit with flats or loafers, dressed up with a cardigan, pearls, and mules, or toned down with a man's cotton shirt or bateau-neck top and flat mules.

Equally versatile are the calf-length, tapered, yet loose-fitting pants that were known in the forties as pedal-pushers. Pedal-pushers got their name during wartime gas shortages, when riding a bicycle became the common mode of transportation, and the conveniently shortened pant didn't get caught in the bike's chains. Sometimes pedal-pushers came with matching tops and turned-up hems.

A variation with a slightly narrower leg that ended just below the knee appeared in the fifties. Called the capri pant (named after the resort island in Italy by the originator of the pant, Emilio Pucci), it was an immediate success. Look for those that are made of ribbed cotton and that have detailing like back buckles and button-down flap pockets, a popular style with Fruit of the Loom, Sears, and designer Johnathan Logan. The shin-baring pants, sometimes known as toreadors or clamdiggers, gave Audrey Hepburn that beatnik appeal in *Funny Face* and exude Jackie O chic when styled with a twin-set and scarf.

Palazzo pants, also known as beach pajamas, are another fantastic find. They're wide-legged, fluid, and comfortable pants that became very popular in the 1930s, and were worn primarily during "leisure" time, over a

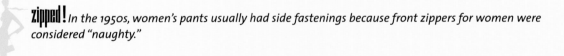

zipped! *In the 1950s, women's pants usually had side fastenings because front zippers for women were considered "naughty."*

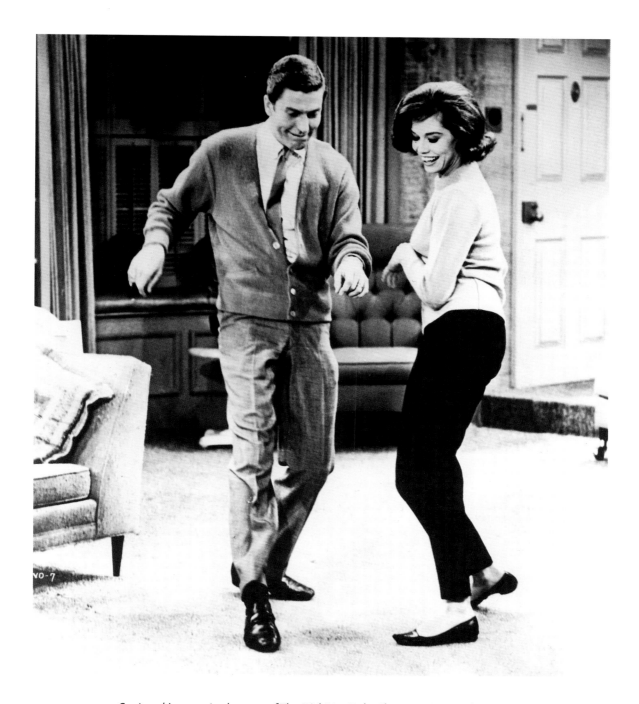

Captured in perpetual reruns of The Dick Van Dyke Show *are Mary Tyler Moore,
in cigarette pants and flats, and Dick Van Dyke in his "at-home" cardigan, doing the Peppermint Twist.
Opposite: Late 1960s palazzo pants with white beaded paisley pattern.*

bathing suit at the beach or on the golf course. Sometimes they daringly made their way into cocktail lounges, with matching tunics or jackets. They epitomized the "American Look," a casual yet elegant attire that reflected the ease of the American woman's lifestyle; a look which designer Claire McCardell helped make the trademark of the American woman.

Their flowing shape, with voluminous legs and draping and loose fit, suits all body types, and can be transformed from a relaxed summer look with a T-shirt and espadrilles to an elegant evening effect with a long tunic or belted jacket, mules, and Bakelite bangles; or with a barebacked halter, clingy wrap top or body suit, a wide belt, and ballet slippers for a sexy night out. Check the "pant" and the "sleepwear" section for them. Some pajama bottoms, although not traditional palazzo pants, will do the trick.

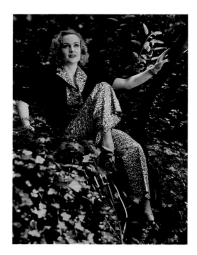

Carole Lombard blends into the foliage in her palazzos and matching top.

Along with palazzos, look for drawstring pants (and long skirts) from the 1940s, another favorite of designer Claire McCardell. Their simplicity, comfort, and versatility regained popularity in the late 1960s and 1970s, when designers turned to Eastern and Asian cultures for inspiration. The pants' free-flowing style was immediately embraced by the free-spirited, free-flowing, and practically gender-neutral look of the hippie generation.

Khakis or chinos are classic vintage buys. Although the original khaki has not changed drastically over the years (see page 89 for more information on the history of khakis), buying a pair of soft, worn-in chinos off a thrift store rack is far more rewarding that going for "this season's" cookie-cutter design, churned out by manufacturers and sold by the millions in chain

jackie oh! *It was rumored that Jacqueline Kennedy once showed up at a top New York restaurant wearing palazzo pants and a long tunic, only to be informed that the dress code did not permit women in pants. With her usual sense of dignity and discretion, she excused herself and repaired to the ladies room, where she removed the pants. She emerged seconds later and sat down to dinner, wearing only the long tunic.*

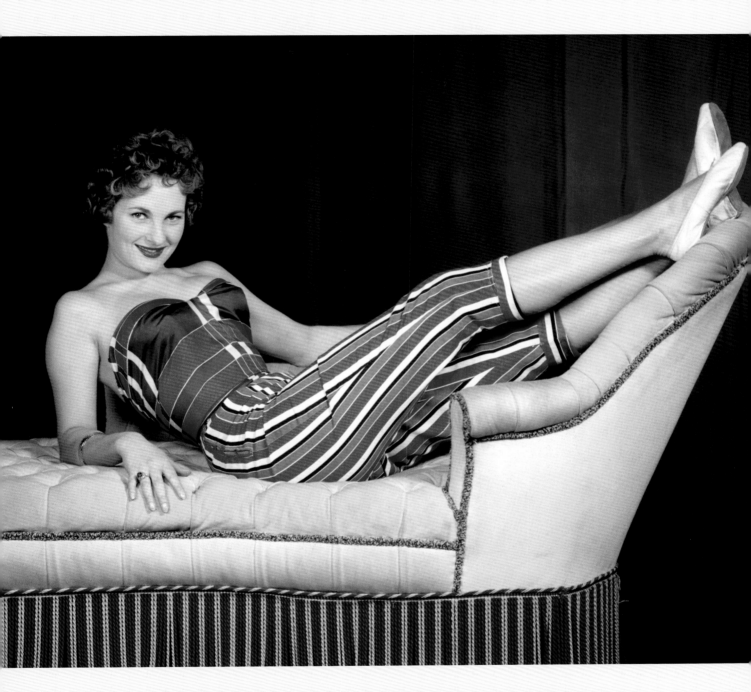

Pedal-pushers aren't just for biking, especially when paired with a red hot bustier (1955).

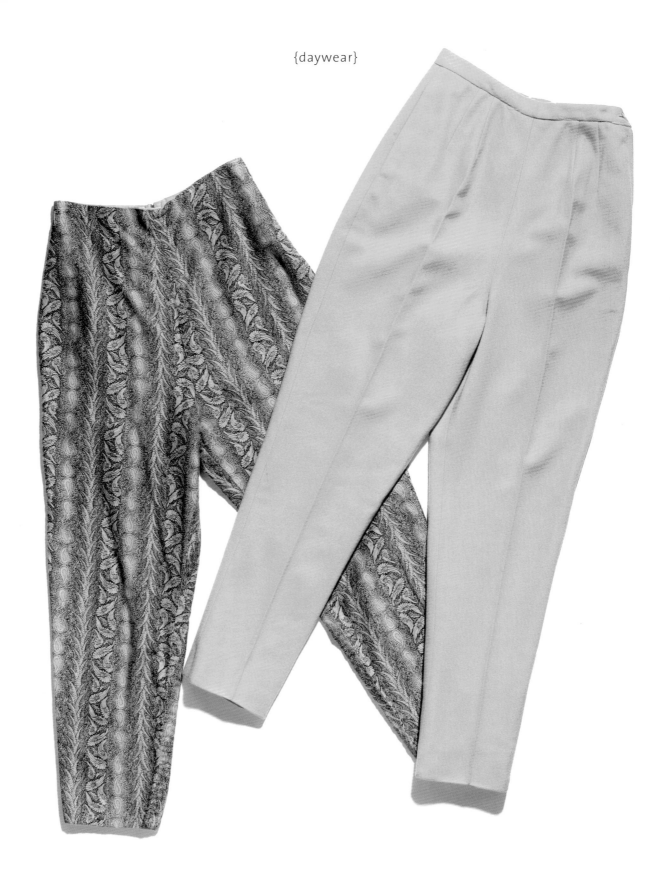

pant particulars

*• If you find a pair of pants you like,
look in the jacket section for its mate. It might be part of a suit.*

*• If the hem is too short, frayed, or stained, you can always lop off the bottoms and make
a great pair of shorts or "highwaters" out of them.*

*• Inspect seams, pockets, buttons, buttonholes,
zippers, linings, and belt loops for tears, frays, and missing parts.*

stores. Each pair of second-hand chinos has a little something special that new ones don't offer—a bit of history, mystery, and certainly more variation in style. Try on the whole lot: side-buttoned, zip-fly, button-fly, pleated, flat-front, cuffed, hemmed, frayed, plain-front, and pocket-front. Remember to forage through the men's and children's sections for additional examples. You can always wear them belted, rolled up, or loosely riding low on the hips paired with a cotton tank or classic man's shirt; slip into them with a chunky sweater, thick socks, and loafers; and even take them out to a casual dinner with a twin-set and animal-print mules.

*Capricious capris: From sizzling pink to taupe paisley patterns, these adorably ankle-baring pants
from the fifties are a daytime natural with mules and a T-shirt.*

{dresses}

Dresses are fun to buy because they constitute an "instant outfit." They're no-nonsense, practical, and easy-to-wear because with just one piece, you're fully dressed. There's no need for mixing and matching with tops or bottoms, no tucking or belting, or fabric confusion. Just a zip or a snap, and then comes the fun part: accessorizing. And fortunately in the world of vintage, there truly is a dress for every body type, for every taste, for every occasion, and for every season. While you're sorting through the multitude of styles, always remember to feel the different textures and to examine the detailing. Dresses from the 1950s are notorious for their attention to intricate finishes and artistry of handiwork: fine stitching, delicate trim

and buttons, precious bows, complex sequin work, embroidery, lace, and appliqués. Dresses from the 1960s, on the other hand, make their own cutting-edge "youth culture" statement through the use of unusual "space-age" fabrics such as Mylar, plastic, PVC, lurex, chain mail, vinyl, rubber, paper, cellophane, and even aluminum foil. They also feature psychedelic prints and all-over patterns.

And let's not forget the classic, simple sheaths and shifts from the same era, the ones in one-tone pastels, white, and cream made popular by Jacqueline Kennedy—made exclusively for her by Oleg Cassini—and topped with Halston's pillbox hats. Early seventies dresses are more about ethnic prints and beads, synthetic jersey, suede or leather trim and fringe, patchwork, and crochet. The fashion of the late seventies celebrates the glitz of disco with rhinestones, spandex, fluorescent satin, lamé, glitter, and polyester. Lots of polyester.

You can never go wrong with an A-line dress. No matter what your body type, the dress's distinctive triangular silhouette, which puts minimal emphasis on the breasts, waist, or hips, just slips right on. The A-line dress was first introduced by designers Christian Dior and Mary Quant in the early sixties, and they were an immediate success. Their shape gave women instant freedom, mobility and versatility, something which the more constructed dress of the 1940s, for example—with its intricate padding, stitching, boning, and structuring (typical of Christian Dior's "New Look")—could not provide. The A-line can glide from day to evening with a different set of heels, from classic elegance with a cardigan casually thrown over the shoulders, to a daring "mod" look with a pair of calf-defining go-go boots and geometric earrings.

The original shift dress, a slim-fitting garment that barely covers the knee and skims the curves of the body, is another classic that easily makes the transition into today's wardrobe. In the late fifties and early sixties, shift dresses were popular in thick stripes, pop art designs, and floral patterns (especially large roses), and were usually made from textured fabrics with substantial weight, like brocades and knits, for better draping. Today's version of the shift dress usually comes in a solid color and is made from a lighter fabric. The vintage version is definitely more fun. Pair one with knee-length boots and tights, or with heeled slingbacks and a vintage "poured-glass" brooch for afternoon cocktails.

The printed day dress from the 1950s—the kind Lucy wore in *I Love Lucy*—is still an easy find in today's increasingly competitive vintage market. That's because advances in manufacturing and mass-production techniques after the war sent the ready-to-wear industry booming. There were many more of these dresses made available then, so naturally they are

Flanked by two typical linen shift dresses from the sixties, one with a floral pattern and the other with a pop-art design, this 1960s, signed Emilio Pucci short-sleever is a collector's dream.
Opposite: A classic day dress from the sixties, with embroidered flower and leaf pattern.

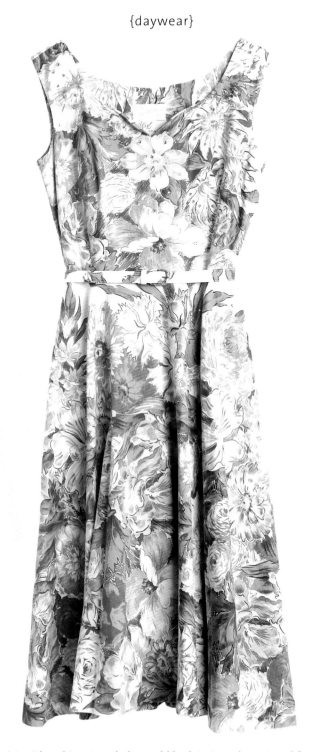

This cotton floral shirtwaist with a rhinestone belt would look just as elegant and feminine today with a pair of slingbacks and a cardigan draped around the shoulders, as it did almost sixty years ago.

easier to find today. These sweet, summery frocks exude the spirit of post-war détente and prosperity, and are easy to spot in a crammed thrift shop or flea market. In cotton, nylon, rayon, gabardine, taffeta, chiffon, and satin, swirling with flowers, vines, leaves, and abstract prints, they bloom with bows, small rhinestone buttons, piped trim, thin belts, and flirtatious details. They're a bit fitted in the bodice and flair out at the waist into a full, mid-calf length skirt that is either lined with a stiff under-slip or comes with a detachable one. Some dresses are sleeveless; others have cap or short sleeves, and some have halter tops. They are divinely coquettish when paired with ballet flats and a little raffia purse from the same decade, and stylishly seductive with stilettos and a pashmina shawl.

And of course, you have to have a little black dress, to wear day or night, from morning latte to late lunch, and straight into the cocktail hour and through the evening. The little black dress (that's "LBD" to the connoisseur) is fashion at its most fundamental; versatility at its best, in every decade and in every style. It defies age and cost barriers. It can be sexy or severe, dressed up or played down, stunningly simple or devastatingly effective, sassy and accessorized or serene and somber. It provides an opportunity to exploit simplicity with flair and finesse (a strand of pearls here, a subdued pump there, and a coupe de Champagne perhaps?), or to play up its monochromatic appeal with exuberance and over-the-top fantasy (a rhinestone choker, chandelier earrings, silver mules, a wide-brimmed hat, saucy stilettos, and a feather boa…or two). Most important, look for one that flatters your body type and that is made of

the shirtwaist dress

The fifties also gave birth to the classic belted shirtwaist dress, perfect for either day or evening. Usually designed with wing or standing notched collars and a thin belt, these classic dresses were a must-have throughout the decade. Cotton, nylon, and jersey were popular daytime fabric choices, with rayon, taffeta, and silk reserved for eveningwear. If the dress fabric is in a solid color, it generally means that it has good texture or draping quality. Because the fifties was the decade in which designer fabrics entered the fashion scene, prints of all sorts—from polka dots to artist-inspired abstract designs—were hugely popular. Elaborate beadwork, lace, or rhinestones were also added for extra pizzazz.

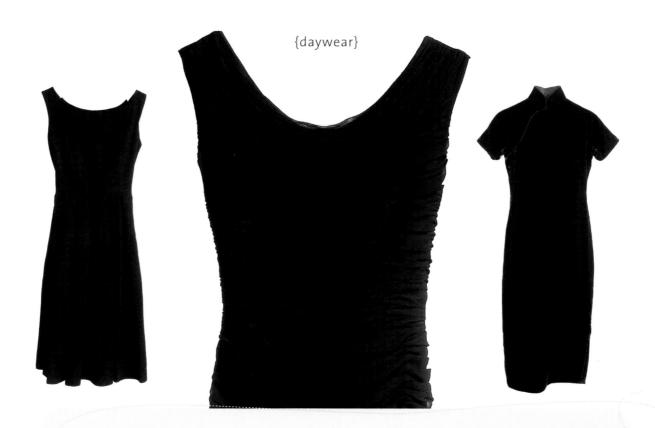

the little black dress

Although many designers want to take credit for the invention of the little black dress, honors go to Gabrielle "Coco" Chanel, who introduced it in the May 1926 issue of American Vogue. It was compared to "Ford's shiny black standardized motor car. Both were sleek and intended to be available for the masses. The little black dress was set to 'become the sort of uniform for all women of taste.'"[3]

1930s: Cut on the bias in satin or crepe, its slender and sleek silhouette drapes Jean Harlowe.

1940s: The hemline gets shorter, shoulders grow bigger, it's draped in fox fur and topped with cocktail hats. Three-quarter length sleeves are complemented by long gloves. Think Joan Crawford and Bette Davis.

1950s: The LBD is longer and fuller, with layers of taffeta and stiff petticoats; it is slim, trim, and shorter when cut as a sheath dress; or loose and chemise-like, a popular design of the late 1950s known as the "sack" dress. (Doris Day in Pillow Talk *(1959) or Jack Lemmon masquerading as a woman in* Some Like It Hot *(1959).)*

1960s: The LBD establishes itself as a fashion icon. Audrey Hepburn as Holly Golightly in a Hubert de Givenchy, accessorized with a cup of coffee and danish, a long black cigarette holder, a martini, a heavy pearl choker, long gloves and a tiara. A strapless number worn by Anita Ekberg in Fellini's La Dolce Vita. *In* Sweet Charity *(1969), Shirley MacLaine flaunts it with a belt, a top hat, and a tattoo.*

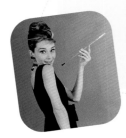

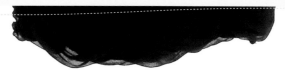

Despite its current cachet, the little black dress has rather grim origins: it was inspired from nineteenth-century mourning rituals during which widows were expected to remain in black for at least two years. Over the decades, however, it has become synonymous with style, grace, and elegance, and has taken on many different shapes and styles, always remaining a fashion staple.

high quality fabric (crepe, wool jersey, silk, or satin), preferably lined.

Then, there's "the wrap." The wrap dress, made famous by American designer and former princess Diane Von Furstenberg, who sold more than five million of them for about $89.00 in the early seventies, has emerged as a fashion icon. Its revival and recent popularity have secured the return of contemporary versions of "the wrap"—including a revised Von Furstenberg original—to the racks of practically every high-end department store and boutique. But the authentic little dress from the seventies, the one made from wash-and-wear soft jersey, the one that bared just a touch of cleavage and was secured by a small bow at the waist, continues to be a regular find on the vintage market. And of course, at a fraction of the cost. Worn by such celebs as Betty Ford, Gloria Steinem, Mary Tyler Moore, Jerry Hall, Aretha Franklin, and Courteney Cox Arquette, it defies age, style, and to some extent, body type.

When it first came out, the wrap dress was an instant hit among career women who wanted the ease and simplicity of one-piece dressing coupled with comfort and femininity. Several versions of the dress (some with collars, others without; some with long sleeves, others with shorter ones) quickly found their way into every woman's wardrobe. In fact, the wrap was such an immediate success that it landed the designer a cover on the March 1976 issue of *Newsweek* magazine accompanied by the headline "Rags to Riches," and a similar article on the front page of *The Wall Street Journal*. Today, its easy-wrap-and-tie style is comfortable, adaptable, practically crease-resistant, trans-seasonal and more important, it's a total knockout. The wrap remains modern and sophisticated for day and slinky-sexy by night, with bare legs and high-heeled sandals or pumps. It's comfortable to travel in and easily packable —rolled up and tucked in a corner of a carry-on, it weighs next to nothing. Just don't be put off by the way it looks on the hanger. You have to slip into it to understand why it's a must-have.

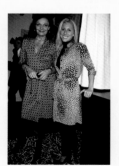

Diane Von Furstenberg steps out in a revival of her own signature wrap dress (1997). Opposite: The little black dress never goes out of style, and these precious jewels from the fifties and sixties only get better with age.

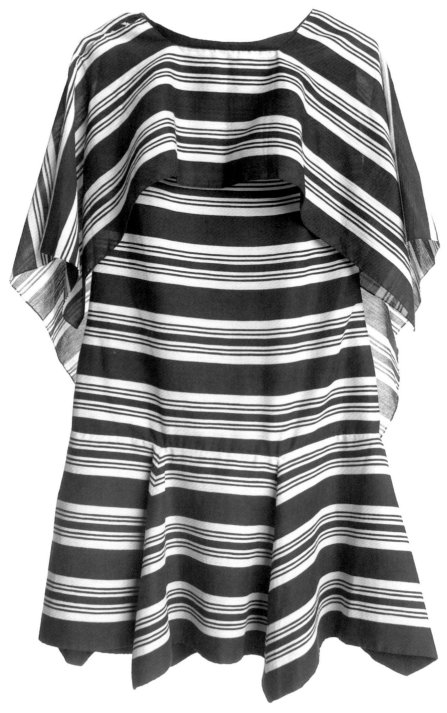

An original Pauline Trigère striped dress with matching cape from the seventies was a find for fifty dollars at a used clothing store; hand-stitching and white daisy appliqués define the neckline of this sweet 1960s light blue linen dress.

{skirts}

Mini, midi, maxi, pencil-slim, A-line, pleated, circular, tiered, swing, flared, full—it all depends on what tickles your fancy, what suits you best, and what hemline you're most comfortable with. Unlike dresses, which have several measurement variables to deal with, including sleeve length, bust size, torso length, armhole width, and back width, the skirt is far more straightforward and negotiable: with a few exceptions, it either fits around the waist or it doesn't. Shortening or lengthening a skirt's hemline (always check for availability of extra fabric at the hem) or moving a button a half-inch to the left

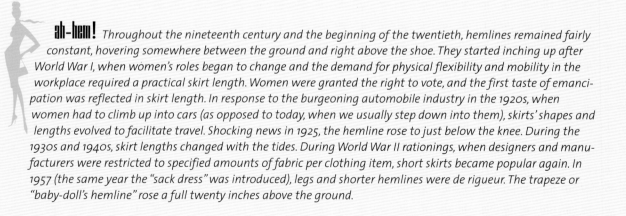

for a little extra room is probably the most of your worries. Still, the skirt has endured more fashion fickleness than practically any other wardrobe staple out there. Since its first major overhaul in the early 1920s, when the skirt parted from its constricting bustles, hoops, petticoats, and crinolines (thanks in large part to Coco Chanel) and opted for a straighter and simpler line, it has shown signs of bi-polarism, specifically when it comes to length. Keeping current with the politically correct hem-length was certainly no easy feat.

The most obvious shock to the system occured

ah-hem! *Throughout the nineteenth century and the beginning of the twentieth, hemlines remained fairly constant, hovering somewhere between the ground and right above the shoe. They started inching up after World War I, when women's roles began to change and the demand for physical flexibility and mobility in the workplace required a practical skirt length. Women were granted the right to vote, and the first taste of emancipation was reflected in skirt length. In response to the burgeoning automobile industry in the 1920s, when women had to climb up into cars (as opposed to today, when we usually step down into them), skirts' shapes and lengths evolved to facilitate travel. Shocking news in 1925, the hemline rose to just below the knee. During the 1930s and 1940s, skirt lengths changed with the tides. During World War II rationings, when designers and manufacturers were restricted to specified amounts of fabric per clothing item, short skirts became popular again. In 1957 (the same year the "sack dress" was introduced), legs and shorter hemlines were de rigueur. The trapeze or "baby-doll's hemline" rose a full twenty inches above the ground.*

in the late 1950s and early 1960s when hems shot up to mid-thigh, the highest in American history. The debate as to who gets credit for the mini still lingers, depending on which side of the English Channel you're on. Some say it was Mary Quant, the British designer who came to personify the Mod look in London. Her daisy logo was soon recognized all over the world and in 1966, she earned the Order of the British Empire by the Queen in recognition of her contributions to British exports and imports. Others, on the other hand, insist that French designer André Courrèges was indeed "father of the mini," as well as the creator of the new "Moon" look, mini skirts paired with silver and white plastic boots and avant-garde accessories. Permanent box pleats became popular then, as well as inverted front and back pleats and reversible skirts.

The late 1960s saw a return to the "maxi," several feet lower than the mini. The maxi and the mini co-existed in harmony, with the same designers producing versions of both. The idea was "anything goes."

The 1970s were more about asserting liberation than anything else. Many hemlines were chucked out altogether in favor of something more unisex like pants or chiffon kaftans. By the mid-seventies, when a recession was beginning to bite, hemlines—and spirits—dropped considerably.

At some point in the mid-nineties, the realization dawned that calf-length skirts are possibly the least flattering look on the planet.

Hello! The new millennium is recalling the mini! According to Nancy Bressner, senior fashion editor at *Cosmopolitan*, "What we've traditionally seen is that anytime a recession is approaching, in response to darker times, designers jazz things up and hemlines go shorter." [4]

A 1970s suede midi skirt with contrasting geometric detail; a classic "H bar C" women's western shirt with snap buttons, front slant pockets, piping, and mother-of-pearl snaps; a pair of women's cowboy boots from the seventies, with stitching and floral overlays. Opposite: Four variations on the 1960s mini.

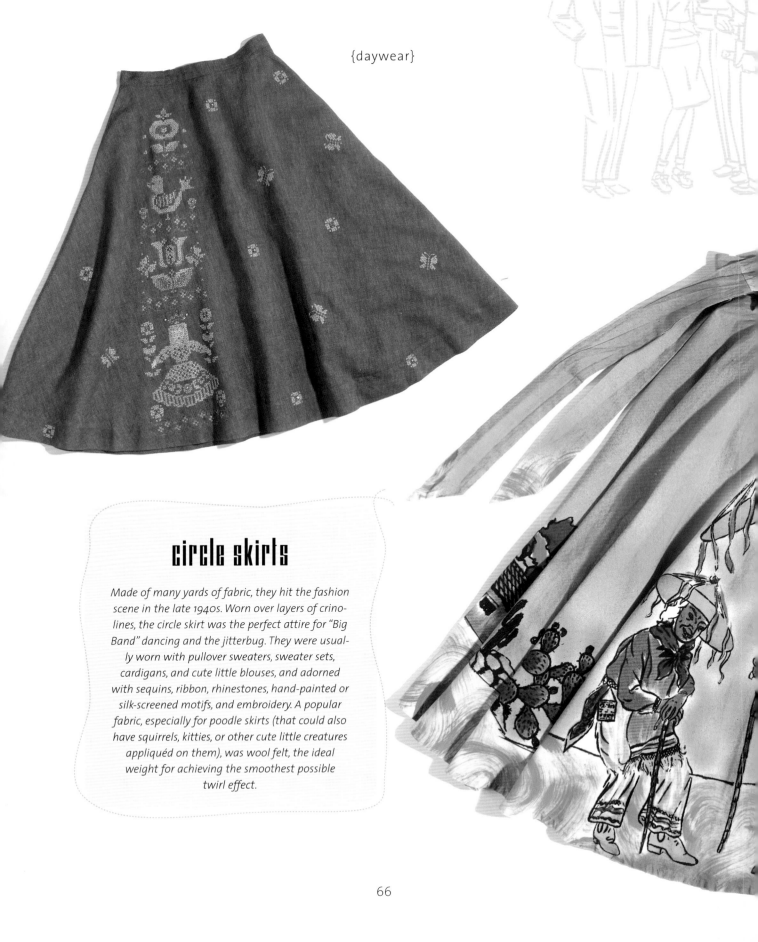

circle skirts

Made of many yards of fabric, they hit the fashion scene in the late 1940s. Worn over layers of crinolines, the circle skirt was the perfect attire for "Big Band" dancing and the jitterbug. They were usually worn with pullover sweaters, sweater sets, cardigans, and cute little blouses, and adorned with sequins, ribbon, rhinestones, hand-painted or silk-screened motifs, and embroidery. A popular fabric, especially for poodle skirts (that could also have squirrels, kitties, or other cute little creatures appliquéd on them), was wool felt, the ideal weight for achieving the smoothest possible twirl effect.

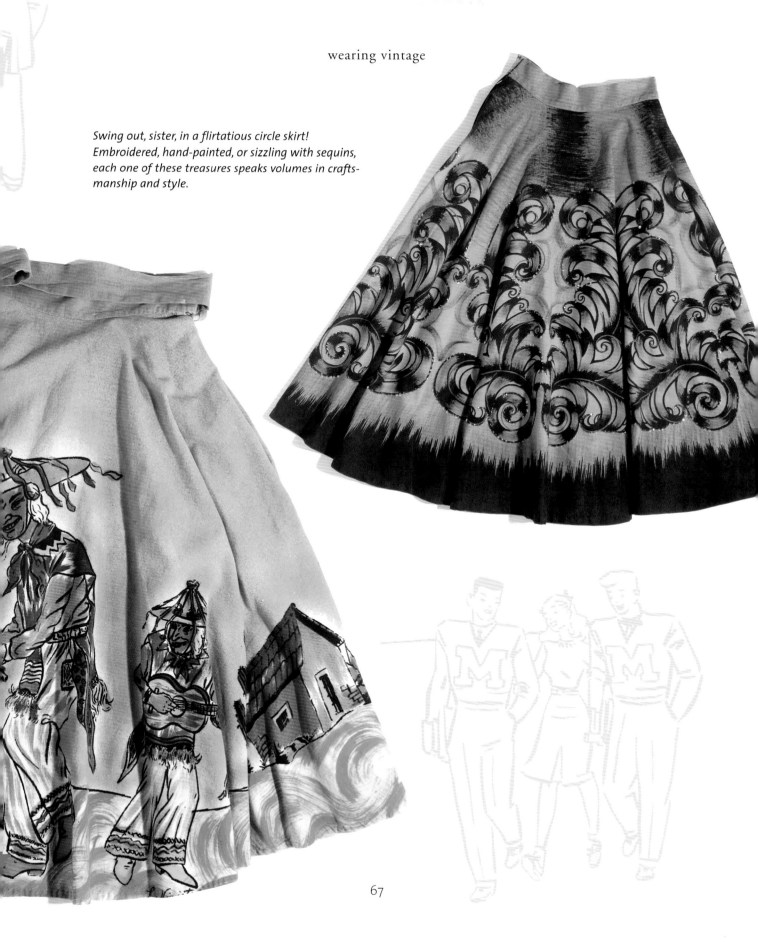

Swing out, sister, in a flirtatious circle skirt!
Embroidered, hand-painted, or sizzling with sequins,
each one of these treasures speaks volumes in craftsmanship and style.

67

{suits}

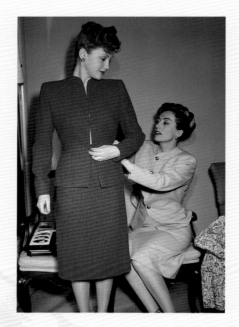

When it comes to vintage skirt- and pantsuits, the hunt can be a bit more challenging. There's always the chance that pants, skirts, and jackets were accidentally separated at some point, never to be reunited; or that if the bottom fits, the top needs some adjusting. Don't despair. Keep an open mind, become friendly with your tailor, and be persistent because you might someday come across a pearl.

Unless you've beaten the "professional pickers" to it, your chances of coming across a Chanel suit from the 1940s or 1950s at your local consignment shop are not the greatest. But you can still strike gold at auction houses and large estate sales. Be prepared to pay as much as $2,000, worth every penny of it, and an absolute bargain compared to the average price of a new one ($5,000). And, you never know what you might inherit from your Great Aunt Francine on your father's side.

suited for success

The thoroughly modern woman of the 1950s had many jobs, both at home and in the workplace. The suit became the popular choice for the career-minded woman, and with the advancement of synthetic fibers, it was easy to wear in and out of the office, and was easy to care for. Similar to men's suitings, women's well-tailored suits were also made of tweeds, wool flannels, and rayon pin stripes. An ad for suits made of Dupont Dacron in 1954 stated: "It's the look you love...from 9 till 5. No wonder so many busy women are finding "Dacron" polyester fiber the beautiful answer for work and play. They love its care-less ways—its delightful habit of keeping wrinkles at a minimum hanging into press overnight, saving inconvenient trips to the presser's." [5]

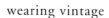

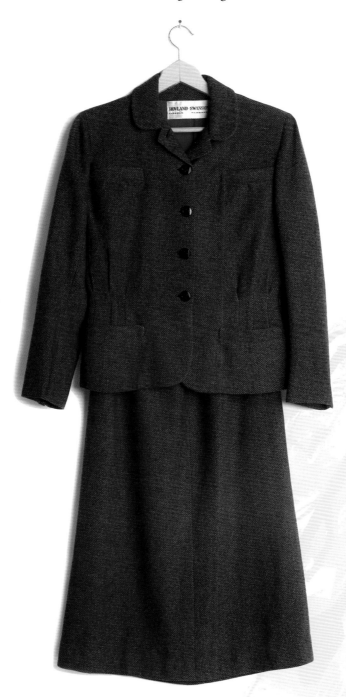

A typical example of a 1940s wool skirt suit, softened by a blouse collar.
On its own, the jacket would look fabulous over a white T, a pair of jeans, and loafers.
Opposite: Well-suited meant big-shouldered in the 1940s. Love the hats!

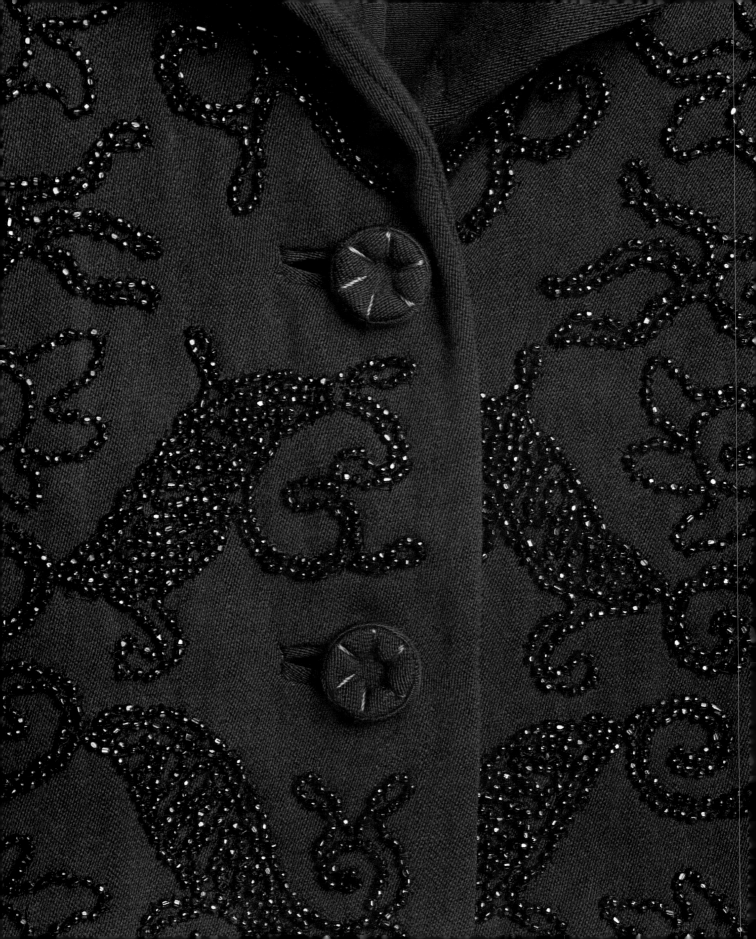

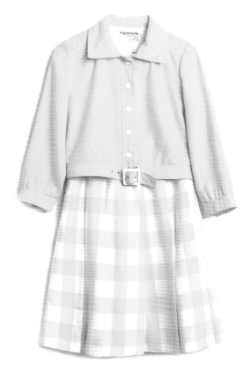

An original 1960s Courrèges suit with trademark white snaps is likely to make every head turn. Opposite: With this much detailing, who needs to accessorize? Aubergine beading and covered buttons glamorize a 1940s jacket.

finding the perfect mate

Remember that thrift shops and vintage stores often separate clothing into categories. Skirts with skirts; shirts with shirts; coats with coats; etc. So whenever you find a fabulous skirt or pant, always check the jacket rack to see if it has a mate.

Take skirt-suits from the 1940s, for example. Highly detailed, nipped-in waistlines, often tied or belted, tapered pencil skirts hemmed from right above the knee to right below, made from silk or heavy taffeta, exquisitely lined and finished (think Joan Crawford)—nothing today even remotely compares to their elegance and style. Or one of the many suit styles from the fifties: slim skirts paired with fitted jackets; boxy jackets teamed up with pleated skirts; belted jackets with straight skirts; or jackets with Peter Pan collars and cuffs.

Try the classic knit suit from the fifties with braid trim and gold buttons; a jersey printed pant-suit from the seventies with wide legs and a tunic-like jacket; or even a man's pin-striped double-breasted suit, cinched tight at the waist, with rolled up sleeves and a simple T-shirt.

{denim}

Buying vintage denim is serious business. Really. Collectors all over the world are willing to pay thousands of dollars to get their hands on a pair of jeans or a jacket from a particular year, with specific tags, seams and buttons, and even with a very specific thread color used for the seams. At a May 2001 auction on the Internet, the oldest known pair of Levi's jeans in existence sold for over $46,000. The one-hundred-and-twenty-year-old pair with an extra pocket riveted on the left thigh was found buried in the mud in a Nevada mining town and was purchased by Levi's Co., who is planning on replicating the old style and selling them new for about $250.

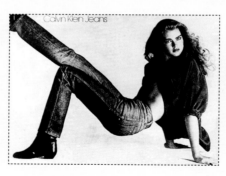

(For details and tips on what to look for when you're seriously trying to find the valuable goods, and for a bit of denim history, see the men's section, page 102). But if you're just looking to buy vintage denim because you happen to like the beat-up look, the worn-in feel, the different styles and dyes, or just because there's no such thing as having too many pairs of jeans and a different jacket for every day of the week, then there is a lot out there for you in vintage land.

And they're all out there: boot cut, straight leg, flared leg, bell-bottomed, tapered, high-waisted, low riders, button-down, zip-fly, stone-washed, acid-washed, "whiskered" (see page 105 for more on that), light blue

genuine jeans

Sex symbol Marilyn Monroe wore them like a glove in the 1961 movie The Misfits, *co-starring Montgomery Clift and Clark Gable. So did French sex-kitten Brigitte Bardot in the 1956 film* And God Created Woman, *in which she paired them with a blouse suggestively knotted under the bust, starting an immediate craze among young women and teenagers on both sides of the Atlantic. And as a result of the (in)famous ad campaign that hurled designer jeans into a multi-million dollar industry, nothing would ever come between Brooke Shields and her Calvins.*

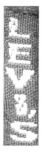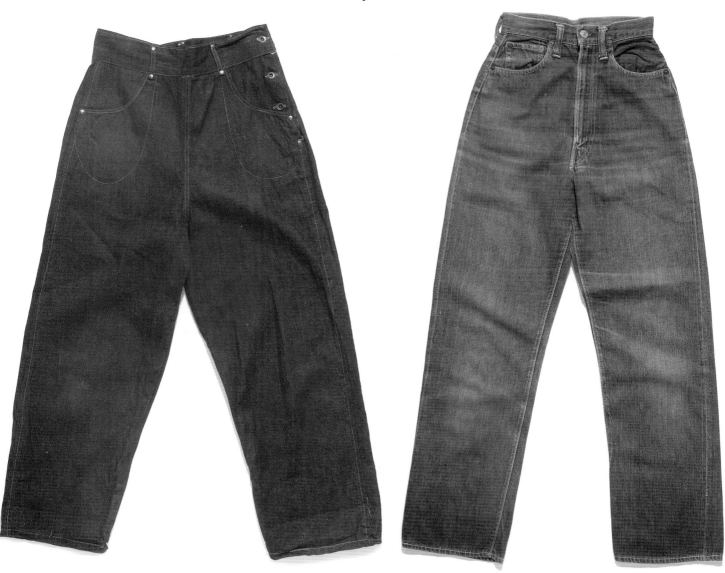

Yes, there was life before "shrink-to-fit" and "stone-washed," and it came with small waists and ample legroom, as in these side-buttoned jeans from the forties (left) and classic high-waisted "Big E's" from the fifties (right). Opposite: Brooke Shields' infamous Calvin Klein ad, in which the nymphet proclaimed, "Nothing comes between me and my Calvins."

true blue! *"Big E's" refers to the capital letter E in the word Levi's on the red pocket tag. The company used these labels roughly between 1945 and 1966 (although some collectors might argue as late as 1971), so the tags read "LEVI'S" instead of "LeVI'S." A pair of Big E's can fetch as much as $1,500 on the vintage market!*

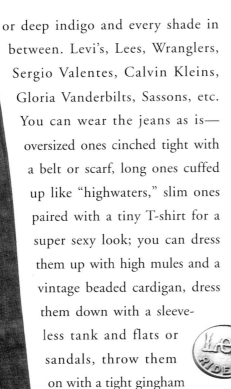

or deep indigo and every shade in between. Levi's, Lees, Wranglers, Sergio Valentes, Calvin Kleins, Gloria Vanderbilts, Sassons, etc. You can wear the jeans as is—oversized ones cinched tight with a belt or scarf, long ones cuffed up like "highwaters," slim ones paired with a tiny T-shirt for a super sexy look; you can dress them up with high mules and a vintage beaded cardigan, dress them down with a sleeve-less tank and flats or sandals, throw them on with a tight gingham shirt (and pretend you're Marilyn Monroe), or you can let them sit low on your hips and just give attitude. You can pair up an oversized denim jacket with a pencil skirt, a boat-neck T and a pair of heels; wear a small one as a shirt with pedal-pushers and sandals, tie one around your waist over a plaid shirt and an oversized pair of chinos. Or, you can just let your imagination go wild. Go ahead, cut them into shorts; remove pockets and put them in unexpected places; shorten them capri style, bleach them, tie-dye them, add pieces of fab-ric or beads, fringe the bottoms, glue rhinestones on them, write graffiti all over them, turn them into a skirt, make them into hot pants, taper the leg, cut off jacket sleeve cuffs and roll them up, sew on patches, or drip paint on them.

One caveat, though. Before you even think of approaching a piece of vintage denim with anything that remotely resembles a sharp object, make sure that what you have is not rare and valuable. Because, once you start slicing, dicing, and julienning—even if it's the tiniest bit—then you've just thrown your around-the-world vacation money or the deposit on your new beach house right out the window. The slightest change to a true collector's vintage pair of jeans or jacket renders it worthless. For more information refer to "Jeans' Genes: What to Look for in Vintage Levi's," page 104.

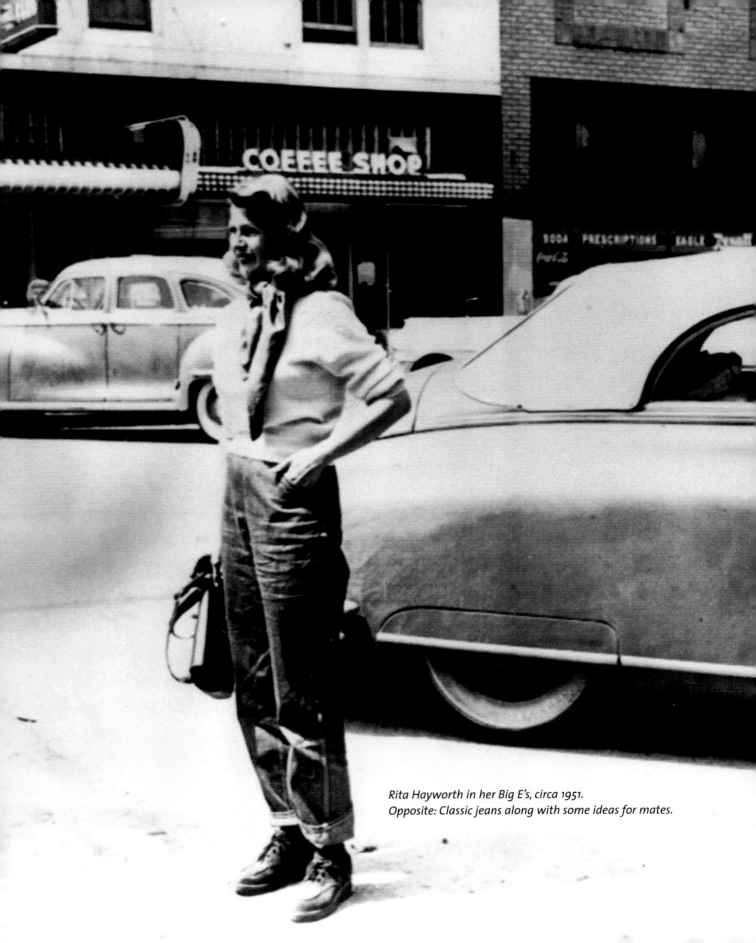

Rita Hayworth in her Big E's, circa 1951.
Opposite: Classic jeans along with some ideas for mates.

{tops, tops, & tops}

Chances of spotting a 1960s Pucci blouse in a consignment shop or thrift store these days are pretty slim. Your best bet for getting ahold of one of these original signed beauties (Emilio Pucci's signature appears in the corner of the shirt) is at an auction house or large estate sale. Nevertheless, you never know what you can dig up at the local flea, so keep your eyes peeled. What you are more likely to encounter, though, are Pucci imitations or rip-offs in similar psyche-delic fabrics but with no-name labels. And if it's more the "look" that you crave, and are willing to compromise a bit on quality and authenticity, these little copies will do the trick. A Pucci-esque shirt or tunic over a pair of white jeans and flat sandals for an afternoon picnic is positively divine, authentic or not.

Then there's always the classic, long-sleeved

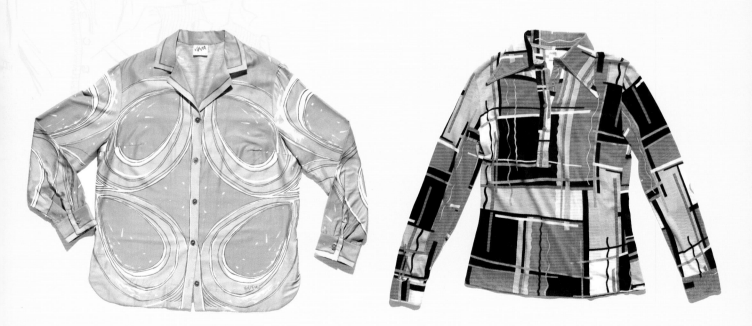

These classic blouses transform basic wardrobe pieces into one-of-a-kind outfits. The 1960s Vera blouse on the left cost about $12 at a thrift shop, and looks great worn as a jacket with rolled-up sleeves over a narrow T and slim pants. The 1970s "Einhorn" makes a splash over a tailored black skirt or pants.
Opposite: Pucci print fabric was signed all over with the designer's first name.

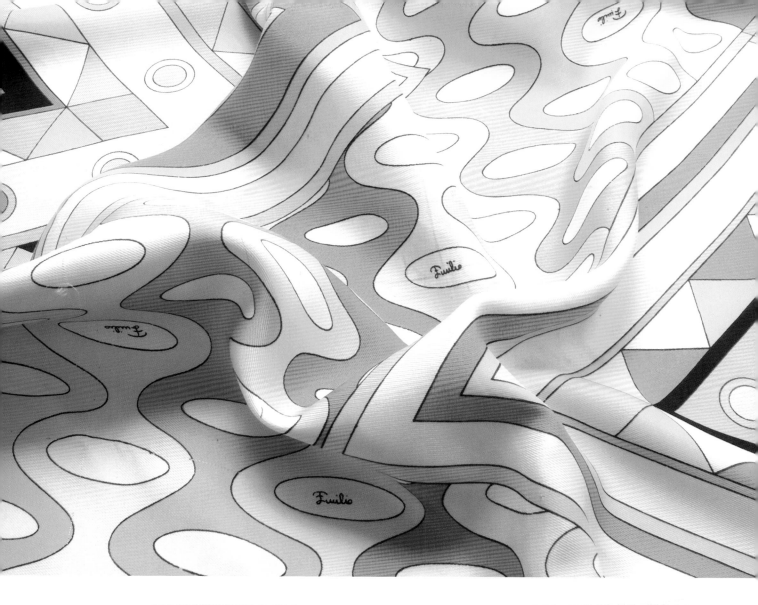

pulsating prints

In part, the psychedelic revolution of the 1960s grew out of the underground drug culture of hallucinogens such as LSD, which was then readily available and inexpensive. The "trips" inspired a technicolor movement, whose impact was particularly felt in design and music. Strong patterns, bursting colors, violently clashing ones that glowed in the dark, vivid greens, oranges, yellows, pinks, and purples made their way into virtually every form of graphic and decorative art. Emilio Pucci, formally known as The Marchese Pucci di Barsento, created some of the most innovative prints reflective of this period. His shirts, dresses, and pants in wildly colored and complex heraldic-style patterns became instant status symbols among the fashion cognoscenti.

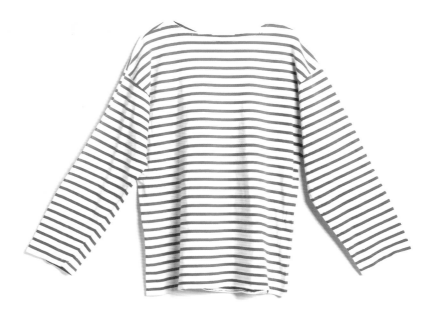

*From French sailors to artists **extraordinaire**, the Breton T has adorned many famous personalities including Pablo Picasso, Audrey Hepburn, and Jean-Paul Sartre.*
Opposite: Designer Jean-Paul Gaultier, with Demi Moore at his side, sports his trademark Breton T after a showing of his haute-couture collection in Paris.

striped blue-and-white cotton boat-neck sailor's T, the Breton shirt, the signature uniform of sorts for French couturier Jean-Paul Gaultier. (Chances are, whenever you see a picture of him on the runway or off, he's sporting one.) It also served as an inspirational muse to Pablo Picasso, Audrey Hepburn, Jackson Pollock, and Tennessee Williams. The original ones were made in the port of Quimper, a maritime town in western Brittany (France), and officially became part of the French sailor's uniform. Since the thirties, however, when Saint Tropez and other Riviera resorts started enjoying a new wave of popularity, the Breton T has sailed from undistinguished workwear to iconic fashion item. It was typically worn tucked into duck bell-bottom pants, which were belted with a silk sash, and accompanied by a pair of long-laced espadrilles knotted above the ankle. Another popular sailor style, particularly for men, featured the Breton T worn with a cravat, under a blazer, over shorts and deck shoes, and topped off with a naval cap. A generation later, the shirt would undergo yet another transformation of identity. After World War II, it re-emerged as "a badge of avant-gardism and youth rebellion in the intellectual ferment of post-Liberation Paris" worn by existentialist Jean-Paul Sartre and avant-garde filmmaker Jean Cocteau.

the many other lives of the breton t

• In the 1950s, Picasso was famously photographed in his.

• In 1965, Edie Sedgwick paired it with black tights for her role in Andy Warhol's Kitchen.
Lou Reed and John Cale of the Velvet Underground, a group originally styled and produced by Warhol,
were regularly photographed in theirs.

• In Warhol's 1971 film Ciao! Manhattan, *Edie is surrounded by elements of her happier past,*
including a Breton T which spills over from an open drawer.

• In 1982, Querelle de Brest, *a film which chronicled the exploits of a seductive homosexual sailor and murderer,*
featured actor Brad Davis in a long coat, Breton T, and sailor's cap.

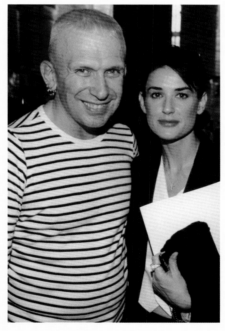

Then in America, and via Hollywood, the Breton T-shirt became a favorite. In the 1956 musical *Funny Face*, Audrey Hepburn wore a black turtleneck sweater and ski pants, plus, of course, a Breton T. In the late sixties, Andy Warhol took an extreme liking to it, sporting it under a jacket, with a pair of black jeans, and with his Centenari & Zenelli "Beetle Boots." In May 1965 he filmed *Kitchen*, starring model Edie Sedgwick, in which she wore the trademark Breton T and black tights. This look has remained a shorthand for Warhol's sixties style, but it was almost instantly iconic.[6]

If you see one, snatch it up quickly. You can't go wrong. It doesn't matter if it's ten, twenty, or fifty years old, the style hasn't drastically changed. The adorable little striped boat-neck, coupled with capris, jeans, cropped khakis, white pants, sexy shorts, or a summery little skirt with espadrilles and a scarf (Hermès or not) loosely tied around the neck exudes freshness and the ultimate in joie de vivre, Mediterranean style.

{men's daywear}

"The problem you're likely to encounter after a zip through your local flea or second-hand shop is one of closet space shortage."

The vintage market for men's clothing has recently started to boom, in large part because there's so much more available out there now than ever before. Some dealers speculate that it's because the attention to men's fashion is a fairly recent phenomenon, brought to the fore in the early 1970s by designers like Ralph Lauren and Giorgio Armani, and ultimately propelled into the spotlight by movies such as *American Gigolo* and *Saturday Night Fever*. Others say that because the style of men's clothing has never been quite as diverse and as seasonal as women's, there was never as much to go around in the first place; that men in general bought fewer clothes and pretty much wore out whatever they had; or that it's a well-known fact that men have always had less closet space than women. Regardless, all of that has changed. While the contemporary man is continually expanding his fashion horizons, he is, for the first time, exploring the past for inspiration and style, for classic pieces, and for just plain old comfort and fun.

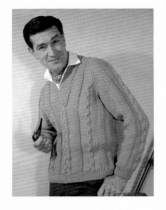

Cable knit can be cool, as in this 1950s long-sleeved sweater worn with a cravat.

fifties sportswear shirts

In the 1950s, when consumers were becoming increasingly "leisure conscious," sportswear became big business. Although the basic dress shirt and the button-down remained popular, a new breed of shirts—sport shirts, longsleeve or short—was hatched. Designed with two-way medium-to-long sport collars, to be worn either open or closed, their double front pockets were either flap or button-down patches. Some shirts had button-shield fronts with elastic waistbands, others had angle zippers and diagonal zipper fronts. The color spectrum included maroon, navy, light blue, light green, salmon, pink, navy, and gray. Two-toned combinations were also popular, with the body of the shirt in one color and the collar, cuffs, and pocket flaps in another. Fabrics of choice were rayon gabardine, cotton, and cotton blends, cotton crinkle crepe, wool flannel, rayon blends, silk, printed madras cloth, cotton mesh, and acetate. In the late fifties, Marlboro Shirt Company launched its "Panel-Rama" style of shirts with a wide horizontal stripe or panel across the shirt for a broader look, or a vertical one for a taller look.

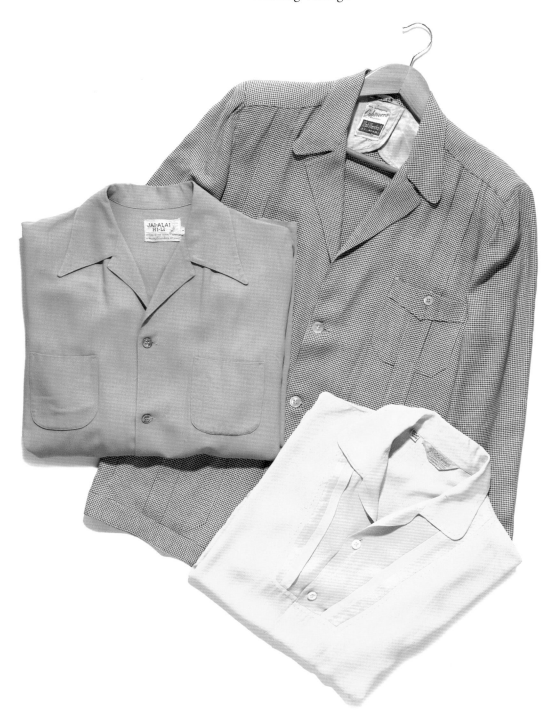

These funky fifties shirts, featuring classic collars and front patch pockets, are as versatile as they are colorful.
Wear them tucked in or let them flow loosely over a T-shirt and jeans for casual flair.

{shirts}

Shirts are very easy to find on the vintage market, and the variety is beyond endless: under one roof, there's everything from basic dress shirts to sports shirts, pullovers, Hawaiian shirts, polo shirts, short-sleeved shirts, long-sleeved ones, flannels, button-downs, and those with stand up collars, pointed collars, continental collars, gaucho collars, curved collars, blunt-point collars, or no collar at all. And then some. Vintage shirts are outrageously cool and add flair and style when paired with any basic pant (Spiegel made some pretty unusual-looking shirts in the 1950s that had collars with side-, back- or no buttons), others are right out of Mr. Roger's Neighborhood, and others might be featured in *GQ*. But be forewarned: The problem you're likely to encounter after a zip through your local flea or second-hand shop is one of closet space shortage.

 man at his best! *Face it. Contemporary style in men's sportswear tends to be, well, style-less. So to avoid looking like every Tom, Dick, and Harry, think Cary (Grant), Robert (Mitchum), early James (Bond), or, yes, even Kramer, and head for vintage shops where you stroll through the eras until you find one that suits you best.*

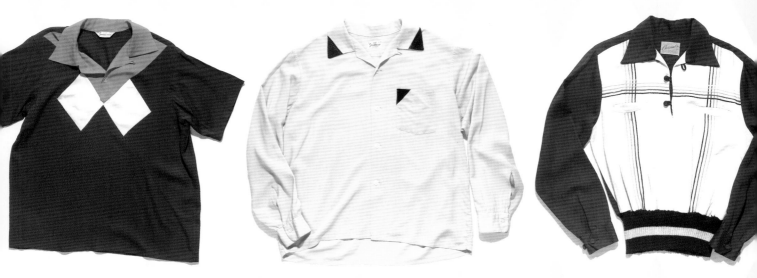

Bored with the old button-down standby? Tired of looking like everyone else at the barbecue? Then pick up one of these fifties gabardine shirts at your local flea. Notice the attention to detail, especially the ribbing and stitching on the pullover on the right.

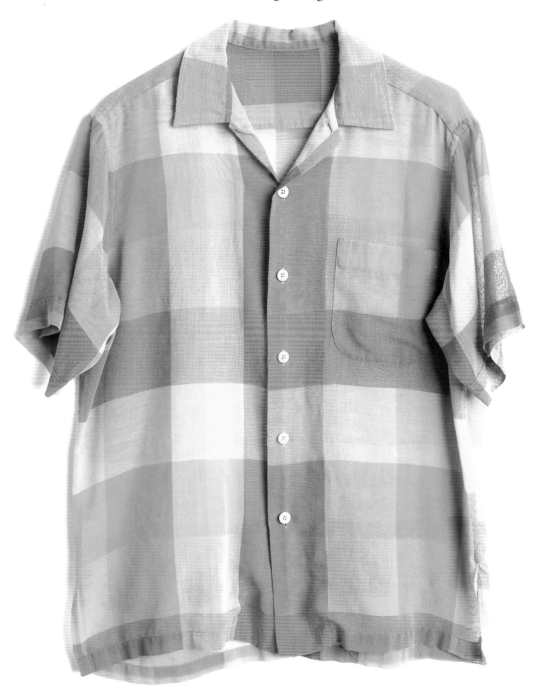

*Play in plaid! Fifties shirts like this one are back in vogue, thanks in part to television's favorite "hipster-doofus,"
Kramer. This lightweight, short-sleeved standard is finished at the hem so you can let it all hang out.*

{hawaiian shirts}

Whether their flamboyance conjures up images of tiki torches and poolside lounging with a large umbrella cocktail (or two), or whether they make you positively wince or wish you were an extra on *Hawaii Five-O*, vintage Hawaiian shirts are such a sizzling collector's item than you simply can't afford to pass them up. Although Hawaiian shirts have gone from laughable to collectible, aficionados are convinced that in a few more years they'll be hanging in museums.[7] For example, a rayon shirt with ukuleles, pineapples, and tropical fish that sold under two dollars in the 1930s can fetch up to $3,000 in today's domestic collectors' market, and probably even more in Japan.

Aloha! This Catalina Hawaiian shirt offers comfort and durability—you'll want one for every day of summer.

But even if the shirt hiding at the bottom of the bin that you salvage for a few dollars doesn't turn out to be a ticket to the bank (poor condition? too new?), you couldn't possibly be in better company wearing one. Serious Hawaiian shirt wearers are men of style and elegance, and they include Tom Selleck, Steven Spielberg, Quincy Jones, and Bill Cosby. Replete with shimmering silk-screened hula dancers, bright and colorful rows of tropical flowers, fields of sugar cane, swaying palm trees, and golden sunsets, these shirts exude an over-the-top yet self-conscious tackiness that is, yes indeed, absolutely charming. Couple them with comfy khakis or a pair of old jeans, kick back, and let the vacation begin.

The forerunner of the Hawaiian beauty was a boxy, printed shirt made with Japanese fabric by small tailor shops in Hawaii in the 1920s. Koichiro Miyamoto, a Honolulu dry goods store owner born in America and raised in Japan, was one of the first to manufacture them, using silk, broadcloth, and rayon. As the tourist trade developed in the late 1920s, a demand for the island's memorabilia grew with it. Tourists and sailors were taking the native shirt home as a souvenir, and pretty soon, the shirt was mass-produced. It gained even more

hunting hawaiian

Look for:

• *Rayon, which is an indication that the shirt might have been made between 1930 and 1955. Introduced by DuPont in 1924, rayon held dyes well, produced clear, sharp patterns, and was stronger than silk. After the mid '50s, Hawaiian shirts were primarily made out of cotton, which were stiffer and didn't hang as nicely as rayon.*

• *A crisp, complex design (newer shirts are less brash in color and simpler in design).*

• *Double stitching on the seams.*

• *Long points on the collar.*

• *Fabric that lines up on the pocket lines.*

• *Horizontal button holes.*

• *Coconut, shell, or wooden buttons, an indication that the shirt was most likely manufactured between 1940 and 1960.*

• *Unique prints with background colors of black, bright blue, red, or yellow. In the 1950s, some Hawaiian shirts were printed on the inside out, with boldest colors on the inside of the shirt.*

• *Labels with miniature island scenes, volcanoes, palm trees, flowers, pineapples, or surfers: Duke Champion Kahanamoku, Kaehaeha, The Kahala, Aloha Tailor, Specially Ruth Made, Andrade, Aloha Shirt Created by King-Smith, Waikiki Fashions Made in Honolulu, Surfriders Sportswear, Pacific Sportswear, Kamehameka Garment Co., and Paradise labels, just to name a few.*

A typical palm tree print is jazzed up with geometric shapes and primary colors on this unusual short-sleeved Hawaiian classic by Lion of Troy. Below: A far cry from Hawaiian sunsets and pineapples, the ocean creatures on this silk beauty from the fifties seem to slither right off the edges.

popularity with World War II, which brought thousands of Americans to Hawaii's military bases, and in 1947, when the Honolulu Chamber of Commerce urged Honolulu city and county governments to pass a resolution favoring the loose, printed shirt as a uniform for its workers during the hot season (June through October). And of course, once Hollywood discovered Hawaii, the shirt was given the ultimate thumbs up. Bing Crosby serenaded in his in *Waikiki Wedding* (1937), Montgomery Clift died in one in *From Here to Eternity* (1953), and Elvis stole more than just a few hearts with his in *Blue Hawaii* (1963).

One of the most sought-after labels in the Hawaiian shirt department is the Duke Champion Kahanamoku label. Duke Kahanamoku was the quintessential Renaissance man. In addition to winning three gold and two silver medals for his swimming exploits in the 1912, 1920, and 1924 Olympics collectively, he flirted with Hollywood on numerous occasions,

playing opposite John Wayne in *Wake of the Red Witch* and rubbing elbows with Henry Fonda in *Mister Roberts* (not withstanding his roles in *Isle of Escape* and *Girl of the Port*), and served nine consecutive terms as sheriff of Honolulu County. And in his spare time, when he wasn't surfing—he was, after all, a surfing pioneer!—he endorsed a line of gorgeous multicolored rayon aloha shirts. Fans of his shirts rave about their blasts of pattern and color, and about the thrill of the cool, smooth fabric against the skin. The Duke Champion Kahanamoku line has been a top seller since 1936.

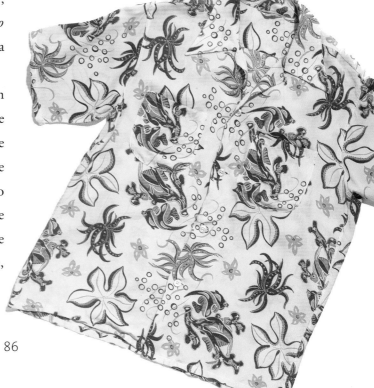

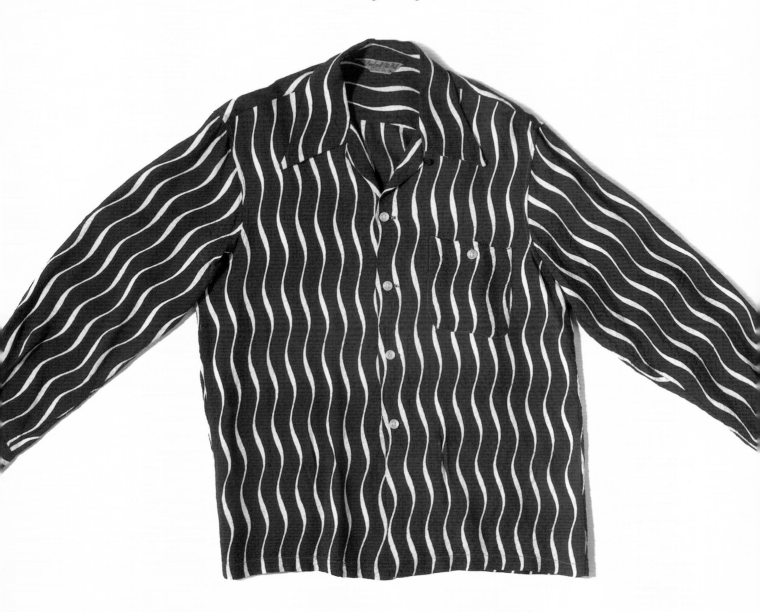

original rayon ! *While many of the original aloha shirts were made of cotton and silk, rayon became the fabric of choice in the 1920s. The vivid colors and intricate designs depicting bits of Hawaiian life—a cornucopia of palm trees, multicolored tropical fish and birds, canoes, pineapples, coconut trees, surfers, huts, sunsets, and hula dancers—came out sharper and clearer on rayon. The fabric was also stronger and less expensive than silk, considered a luxury item at the time. But in the 1950s, a fire destroyed the Dupont factory that supposedly contained "the original rayon recipe," which many claim produced a fabric that was softer than the subsequently produced rayon. And that's when cotton stepped in.*

{bowling shirts}

The bowling shirt, that fabulously fun-colored short-sleeved shirt with a squared-off body and embroidered sponsor or league name, has become scarcer since the mid '80s when the classic made way for knitted polos and T-shirts. Although contemporary manufacturers are trying to replicate shirts that were sported in bowling alleys in the '50s and '60s by imitating their cut, style, and stitching, they rarely have the quality and fit of the originals. And they definitely don't have the karma.

Made from gabardine, rayon, or silk, the typical retro bowling shirt is boxy in cut to allow for a full swing and to ensure a super-comfortable fit. Paired with flat-front chinos or slim '60s pants, the look is laid-back and authentic. Keep an eye out for labels such as King Louie, Nat Nast with the original lion logo, Two Legs Inc., and Hilton. Shirts from the '40s and '50s can be as much as $100, while shirts from the '60s and '70s can range from $15 to $40.

This beautiful example of a fifties gabardine bowling shirt features bowling pin buttons, an embroidered name above the breast pocket, and league tags on the sleeves. Strike!

a sure strike

What to look for in vintage bowling shirts:
• Buttons that match the color of the collar. On some old shirts, buttons are shaped like bowling pins.
• Collars in contrasting colors to the body of the shirt.
A few shirts have the figure of a bowler embroidered on the collar.
• Sleeve hems in contrasting colors.
• Bodies with contrasting front panels, or a different color yoke across the front and back shoulders.
• Embroidered names located above the front pockets; the team logo or sponsor name on the back of the shirt.

{buffalo shirts}

Created in the 1850s, these oversized two-color check shirts (black with red, yellow, blue, white or green) were called "buffalo" shirts because the man who created them also raised buffalo. The cozy flannel shirts with black buttons were originally designed to keep hunters warm and visible to other hunters. Before the mid 1960s, they were largely worn for their intended purpose: outdoor activities. In the late 1960s, however, their sturdy construction, distinctive American look and blue-collar authenticity made them instant campus classics, worn indoors and out. In the late 1970s and early 1980s, hard-core punk bands tied them around the waist. Brands to look for are L.L. Bean, Woolrich, Pendleton, Fruit of the Loom, Lee Union Made, Kenberry, and Eddie Bauer.

This comfy wool Pendleton shirt from the sixties is not all that different from its earliest ancestor, made in 1924 at Pendleton Woolen Mills in Oregon.

pure pendleton

Pendleton Woolen Mills was first famous for its blankets, many of which it furnished to American Indians in the early twentieth century. So synonymous was the company name with trade blankets, based on Navajo designs but not direct copies, that all trade blankets were known as "Pendletons." About seventy-five years ago, the famous men's plaid Pendleton shirt was born. With blue and gold labels reading "warranted to be a Pendleton," the shirts were designed for ranchers, loggers, and sportsmen in the rugged Pacific Northwest who were looking for durability, warmth, practicality, and comfort.

{sweatshirts}

The other thing you should look at, especially with sweatshirts, is the ribbing at the hem and cuffs. Older sweatshirts have a longer or wider rib, and because of wear, hang loosely over the body. Turn the sweatshirt inside out. In older shirts, the cotton is thicker and the reverse side has a fleece-like quality to it. Look for old labels like Hanes, Russell, and Champion (Champion labels from the 1940s and 1950s have a runner on them), and check out how the artwork and logos on labels has changed.

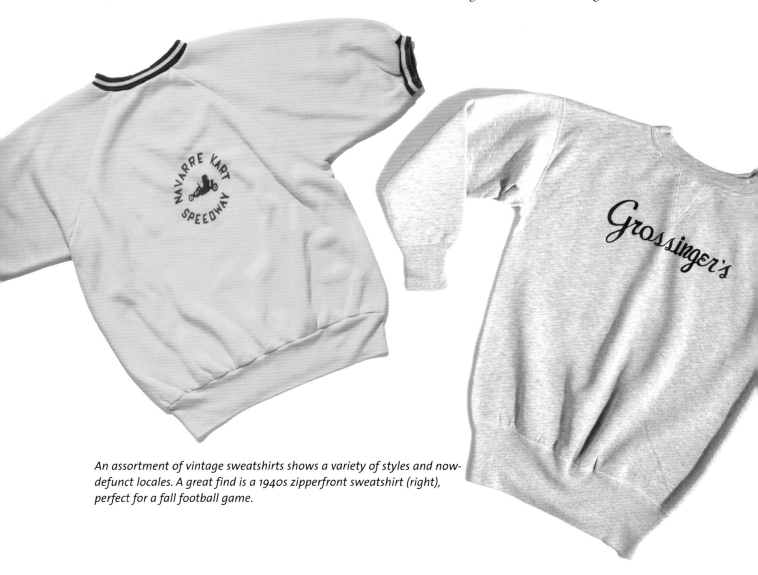

An assortment of vintage sweatshirts shows a variety of styles and now-defunct locales. A great find is a 1940s zipperfront sweatshirt (right), perfect for a fall football game.

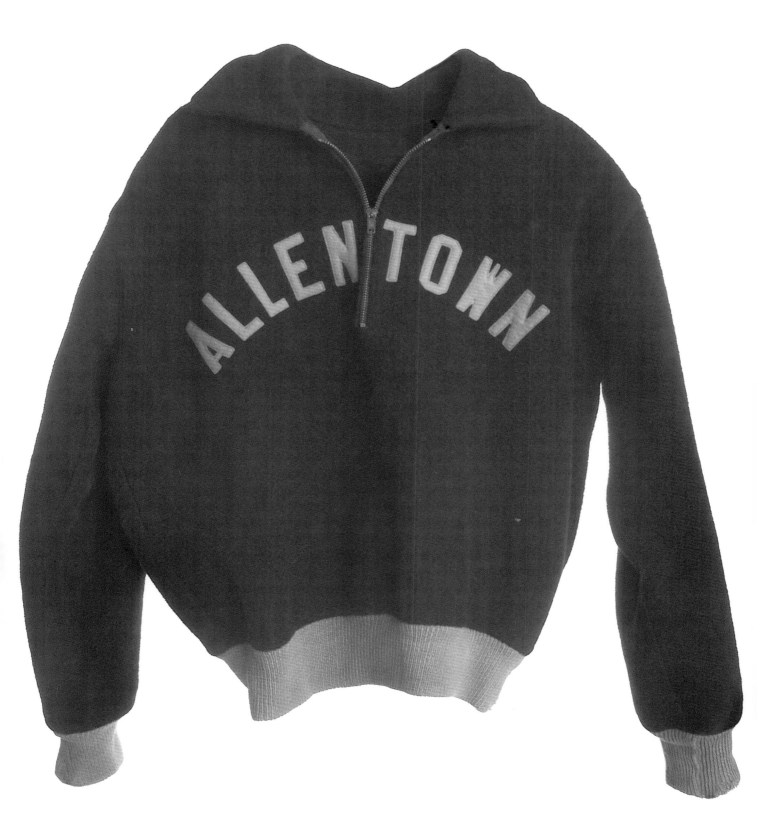

{t-shirts}

The origins of the T-shirt are rather murky. Some say it can be traced back to sailors' uniforms from the 1800s, when they were worn for warmth and protection from scratchy woolen sweaters. Others say the garment originated in the seventeenth century, when longshoremen in Annapolis, Maryland, started wearing collarless, short-sleeved shirts while unloading shiploads of tea. These shirts were less prone to trapping loose tea leaves, which would make the workers itch. And supposedly, "tea" is where the shirt got its name.

Others say that the traditional Ts didn't officially appear until the beginning of the twentieth century, when British Queen Victoria ordered the soldiers to sew arms on their sleeveless undergarments to spare her the sight of underarm hair when they saluted her. Either way, the U.S. Navy adopted the shirt in 1913 as part of the uniform. By the late 1930s, Sears, Roebuck and Hanes were manufacturing the white cotton undershirt by the thousands. It was to be worn exclusively as an undergarment, and sold for about twenty-four cents. The popularity of the undershirt was dealt a serious blow, however, when Clark Gable took off his shirt in *It Happened One Night* (1934), to reveal to Claudette Colbert and the world that he was wearing nothing underneath. T-shirt sales plummeted. But World War II saved the T from its demise as the Navy ordered millions of white ones, the Marine Corps got theirs in sage green, and after the war, the U.S. Army opted for olive drab.

When James Dean and Marlon Brando sported theirs, tight, with leather jacket and jeans in *Rebel Without a Cause* and *The Wild One*, the T took on whole new "bad boy" aura. It became the battle flag of youthful rebellion. Pretty soon, teenagers all over America were shedding their shirts and blouses—much to the despair of their parents—and opting for Ts. In the sixties, T-shirts became a vehicle for self-expression: from political slogans, messages of self-identity, personal feelings, philosophies and protests, to silk-screened or handpainted masterpieces, the T-shirt was in effect a blank canvas for expressing social, economic, political, and personal views. And also for making groovy tie-dyed patterns.

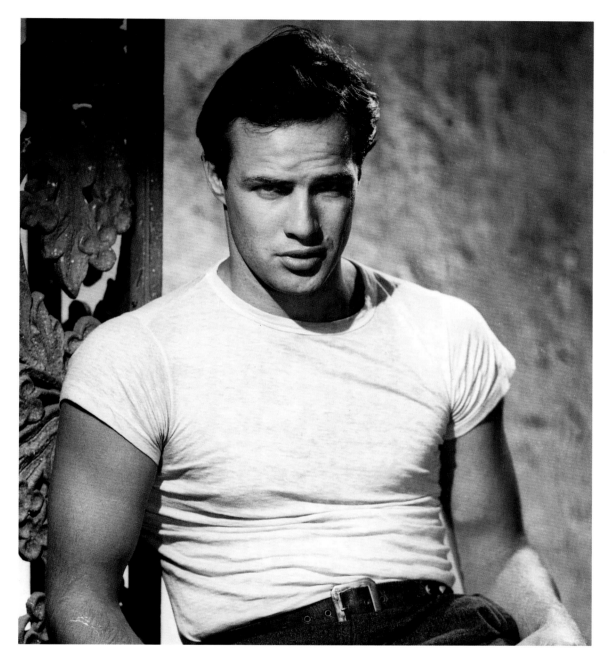

T-shirts never had it so good as on 27-year-old Marlon Brando as Stanley Kowalski, the brutish anti-hero of Elia Kazan's 1951 movie great, A Streetcar Named Desire.

{pants}

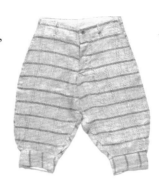

Knickers, trousers, breeches, slacks, pants; bell-bottoms, baggies, elephant legs, straight legs, tapered legs, flared legs; high-rise, low-rise, cuffed, cuffless, tab-waisted, narrow waisted, with an extension band, or without a waistband; plain front, pleated front, with belt loops, sidestraps, back buckles, suspender buttons, or without; flannel, tweed, gabardine, cotton, linen, whipcord, corduroy, denim, knit, stretch, and basically everything from paper to plastic, vintage offers whatever tickles your fancy.

Although these linen knickers might not be your first choice for an afternoon of 18 holes, they certainly dominated the fashion scene at the more elegant resorts in the 1930s.

By the mid to late '50s, the mood was relaxing a bit, and the decade began to sense the emerging fashion influence of European countries, in particular Italy and France. Pants lost their pleats, had a smooth fit and narrow cut, and were tapered to 17 inches at the bottom. Pockets were tilted forward at an angle, finished off with flaps and buttons.

The trim silhouette of the '60s called for an even narrower pant with a low rise, riding on the hip, which *Esquire* noted should be avoided by a heavier man "since a stomach bulging over the top of one's trousers looks most unflattering."[8]

By the mid '60s, slacks made from stretch fabrics were a fashion basic. "Action stretch" provided 30 to 50 percent give and were worn primarily for sports; and "comfort stretch," with 15 to 30 percent give, allowed for freedom of body movement for ordinary daily use. Bell-bottoms, reminiscent of pants worn by college students dancing the Charleston in the 1920s, first appeared as resort wear in 1966. With a multitude of styles to choose from (Baggies? Flares? Bell-bottoms?

having your cake! *In the early twenties, every college man's dream was to go tea-dancing at the Plaza or the Biltmore with beautiful Constance Bennett, the actress daughter of actor Richard Bennett. Dashing in his natural-shoulder suit with wide-bottom trousers, a button-down shirt, striped tie, and argyle socks, he would dance and eat finger sandwiches and cake until dawn. The Ivy League man for whom attending tea dances became an extra curricular activity was known as a "cake-eater," and his 22-inch-bottom suit was called the "cake-eater's suit."*

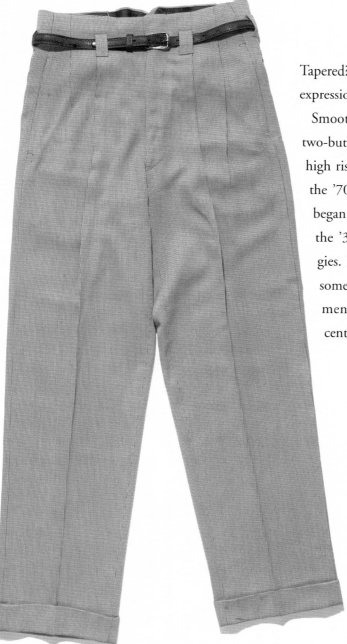

Tapered?), men's fashion became a means of self-expression.

Smooth-fitting, cuffless knitted slacks with a two-button extension waistband or tab closure, a high rise, slanted pockets, and a slight flair was the '70s cut of choice. Pleats at the waistband began to reappear (they had last been seen in the '30s), mainly on elephant bells and baggies. In fact, "there was no question but that some of the most dynamic fashion changes in menswear during the final quarter of the century would begin with pants."[9]

Cuffs, a high waist, pleats, a narrower leg, and low-set belt loops are characteristic of pants from the thirties and early forties. Right: The golf pants here have nifty little tee-holders sewn in above the back pocket.

pantology

• The oldest pair of pants in existence was found at Thorsbjerg, Denmark, and was supposedly worn over 2,000 years ago. The loops on the garment show that it was held in place by a string or a belt.

• A pair of trousers was literally a pair until the fourteenth century, as each leg covering was separate without being sewn together.

• Up until the mid 1920s, close-fitting, heavy-weight knee-length knickers worn with woolen knee socks dominated the fashion scene. They were seen in every fabric, including gabardine, tweed, and a lighter cotton and mohair blend, which was most favored by Palm Beach resorters.

• Knickers grew wider and longer when Ivy League collegians vacationing abroad were smitten with the new fashions worn by students at Cambridge and Oxford universities in England. They were originally sported by the British students to camouflage their undergarments, which had been banned for classroom wear. These "Oxford bags," often worn with a crease in front and in the back, were about 25 inches around the knees and 22 inches at the bottom, and were an immediate success on the American market.

• In 1929, Men's Wear declared that "good taste had knicked the knicker," that the pant was relegated back to the golf course from which it had originated, and that flannel trousers had replaced them entirely.

• By 1935, the resort uniform was a pair of full-cut gray flannel slacks with deep pleats, an extension waistband, side tabs that could be adjusted for comfort and fit, a knitted polo shirt, preferably blue, and two-toned shoes. Bottoms were about 19 to 20 inches wide.

• As a result of World War II Production Board regulations that required conservative use of materials in general, pants were made narrower, and tucks, overlapping waistbands, and pleats were eliminated. Military influence was reflected in civilian wear, as louder shades were replaced with more demure and natural ones like olive, gray, and tan. Eventually, though, man regained his originality, favoring bold stripes, eye-catching plaids, and checks.

• Post-World War II was a period of caution and conservatism: Senator Joseph McCarthy was rabidly ferreting out communists and the U.S. was embroiled in an undeclared war in South Korea. The somber mood was reflected in the understatement in men's fashion. "The man in the gray flannel suit" became the icon for the American man's state of mind. The slim pant had a back strap and buckle but no pleats at the waistband.

Vintage men's pants come in more fabrics, colors, styles, cuts, and sizes than you can imagine. Truly, there is a vintage pant for every occasion and body type.

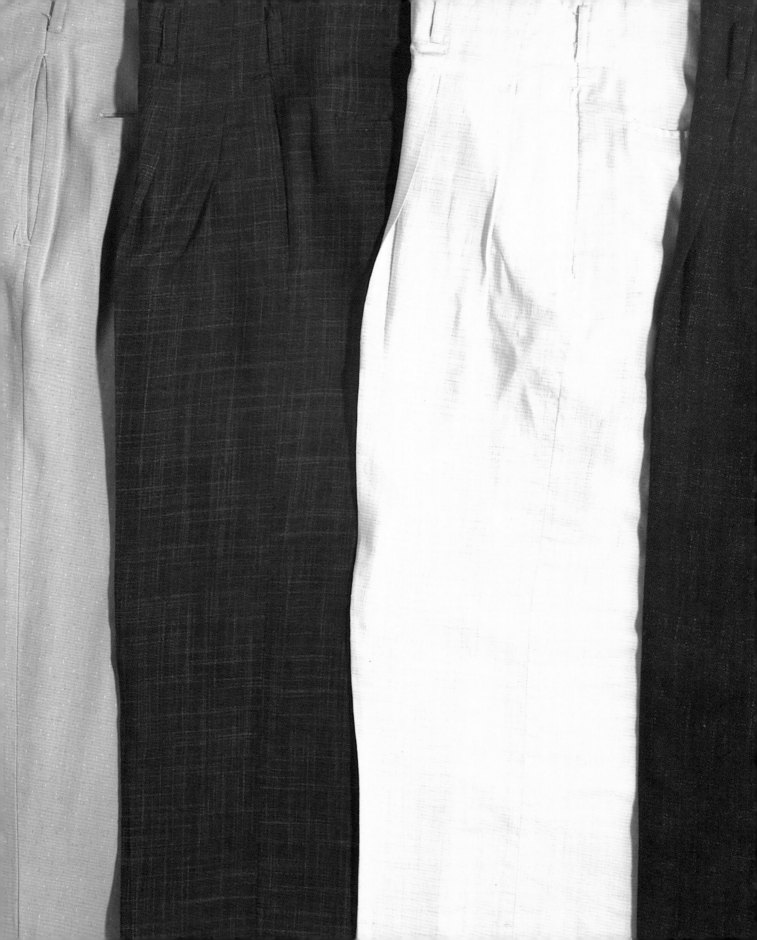

{the classic chino}

A few years ago, The Gap launched a highly successful ad campaign in which more than thirty legendary figures—from Miles Davis, Frank Sinatra, Pablo Picasso, Frank Lloyd Wright, Steve McQueen, and John Wayne to Chet Baker, Jack Kerouac, Montgomery Clift, Ernest "Jack" Hemingway, and Humphrey Bogart—were pictured in a yellowish-brown twill-fabric pant known as the khaki. Today, there's not a man, woman, or child who wouldn't trade in his or her favorite toy for a pair of worn-in, super-soft, extraordinarily comfy pair of chinos. And although the purpose of the ad campaign was to market a current line of khakis, there's no reason in the world why you shouldn't check out the vintage selection first, and find a pair that someone else was kind enough to break in for you.

Legend has it that in 1846, a British army officer stationed in India dyed a pair of cotton pajamas with tea leaves because he was looking for a cooler alternative to his woolen army uniform. The tea leaves gave the fabric a tawny, greenish-beige color and khakis were born. Incidentally,

"Khaki" comes from the Urdu word "kha," which means "dust or earth." The pants got their nickname, "chinos," because until American sportswear manufacturers began making them, they were made primarily in China. In the 1930s, khakis were adopted by the U.S. army for use in uniforms and in the '40s and '50s, the pant gained widespread acceptance across college campuses and universities. Pretty soon, it was the preppy uniform of choice, with sales quickly rivaling that of jeans. In the 1960s, they were hemmed short and referred to as "highwaters" or "floods."

What makes chinos so irresistible is their true versatility. You can wear them loose and wrinkled for a day at the beach, or pressed and creased with a crisp shirt and blazer for a more finished look. You can wear them in the early fall with a T-shirt and heavy cotton cable sweater, and slide right into winter with a cashmere turtleneck. Keep your eyes peeled for army-issue khakis lined with cotton poplin and made of cotton twill that is heavier than that used to make chinos today.

John Wayne was a man's man in cuffed chinos worn Western-style in the 1959 film Rio Bravo.

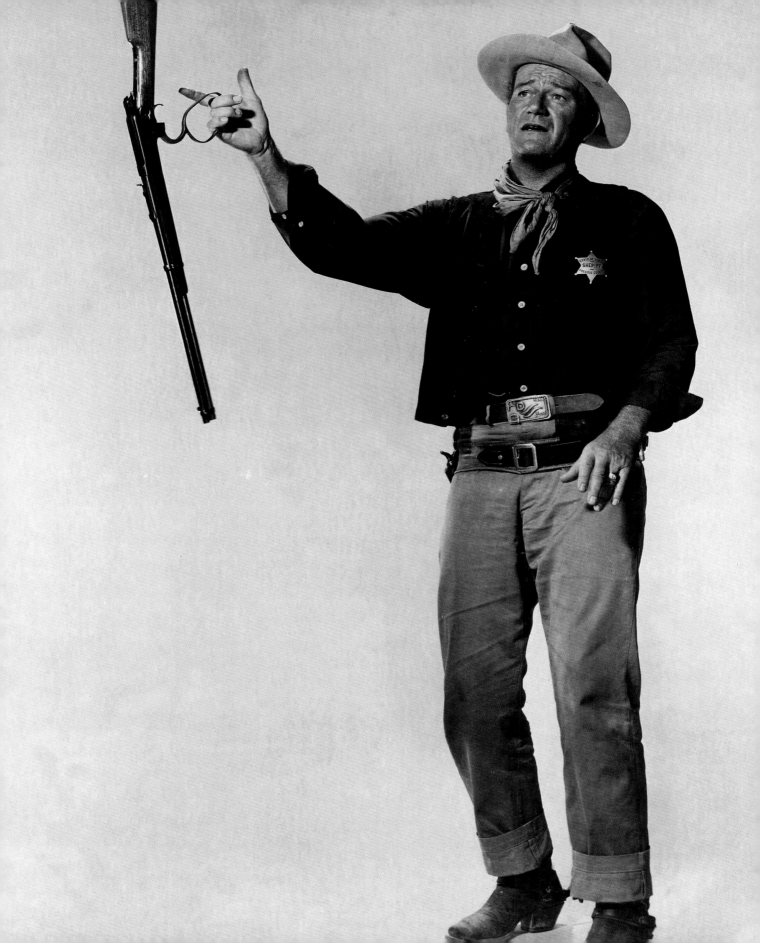

{denim}

Shopping for vintage denim. It just doesn't get any more fun than that. Although, of course, we'll cover what to look for specifically if you want to get the real, authentic, genuine pair of vintage jeans that you could probably sell for thousands of dollars to avid collectors, it's important to remember that the best thing about shopping for vintage denim is that you just can't go wrong. There are so many things you can do with a pair of used five or ten-dollar jeans or a jacket that you just have to go for it. In addition to exercising your creativity—fraying the hems; chopping off the legs to make shorts; splattering paint all over them—and having enough pairs so that you only have to do your wash, maybe, once a month, you can always thrill a sister or a girl-friend, who will relish nothing more than to wear an oversized pair cinched tight at the waist or low on the hips. Same goes for jackets. You can slash off the arms and turn them into vests; remove the collars for a rugged look; or chop off the sleeves mid-length and roll-them up for a short-sleeved version.

Shopping for vintage jeans first became popular when Levi's were only available as "shrink to fit." (Remember sitting in a bath of cold water to get them to shrink?). It was always a tough call to figure out how they would fit and look once they had shrunk. With a used pair, the work had already been done, the fabric had already faded, and there were few surprises when you took them out of the dryer. Today, there's another reason why people are shopping for old denims, on top of the comfort and practicality factors.

jackets

Vintage denim jackets have become so valuable that they are often refereed to as "denim gold" or "blue gold." Look for silver rather than copper buttons and a single front pocket. Watch for pleated folds on the front, discontinued in the late 1960s. Pre-1940s jackets had a buckle on the back. A "Second Edition" vintage Levi's jacket can sell for about $2,000; an indigo-dyed vintage Lee for about $1,100; and a "First Edition" cowboy buckle-back Lee jacket for about $6,000.

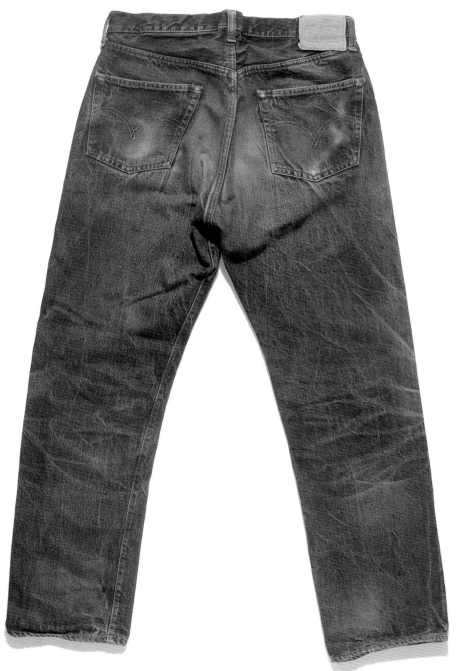

A pair of perfectly preserved late 1940s "Big E's." The ultimate find.

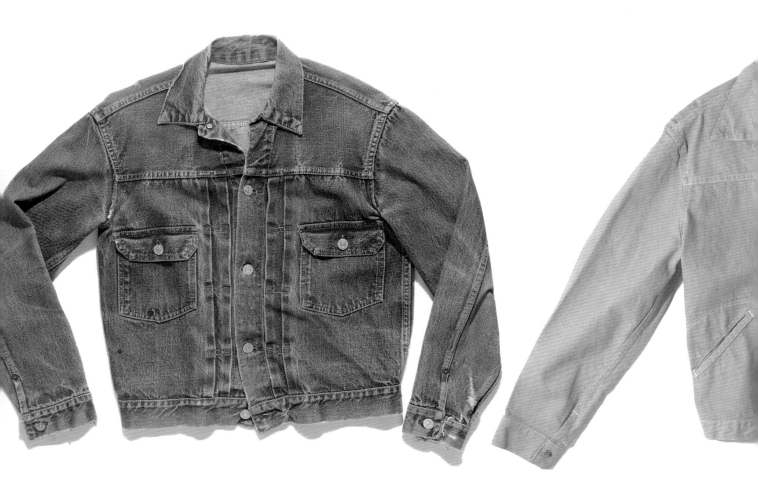

great moments in denim history

1853: Levi Strauss arrives in San Francisco and opens a wholesale dry goods business, targeting primarily American gold prospectors.

1872: Jacob Davis invents the process of adding rivets to the corners of men's pockets and joins forces with Strauss to patent their invention and the "waist overall."

1873: The jean jacket is created as a durable work blouse for gold rush miners in the Wild West.

1890: Levi's assigns its first lot number to manufactured products. "501" is the lot number assigned to copper-riveted overalls.

1919: The Saturday Evening Post runs the very first ad for Lee jeans.

1922: Belt loops are added to overalls, but suspender buttons still remain.

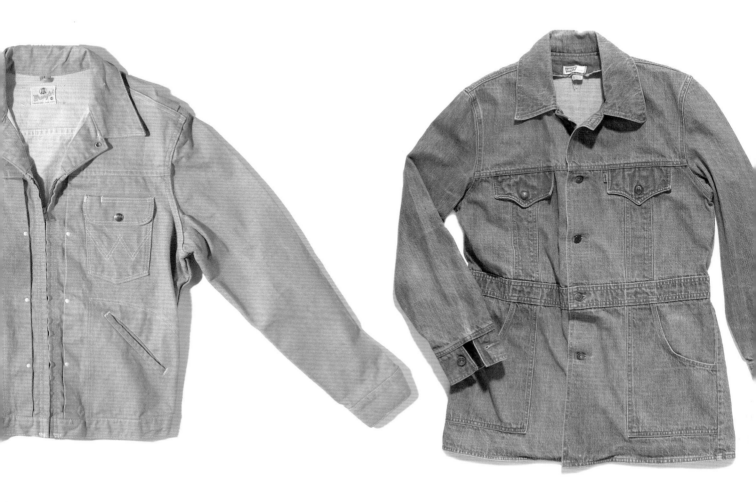

A selection of rare denim jackets includes a 1950s second edition Levi's jacket with two pockets and a big E on its red tag (as opposed to first-edition jackets from the 1940s, which have only one pocket); a collectible 1960s zip-front baby blue Wrangler with vent pockets; and a hip-length 1970s Levi's jacket with deep front pockets.

1936: Levi's "Red Tab" is placed on the right back pocket of waist overalls. LEVI'S (in all capital letters) is stitched in white on it.

1937: Changes are made to waist overalls to conform to rules set by the War Production Board for the conservation of raw materials. The back cinch and the crotch rivet (permanently discontinued in 1941) are removed to save fabric and metal.

1947: Wrangler designs its first pair of jeans. Designed by professional cowboys for professional cowboys.

1954: A zippered version of the waist overall is introduced.

1955: James Dean becomes a jeans icon in films East Of Eden and Rebel Without A Cause.

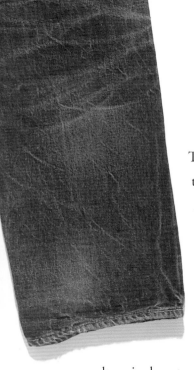

They're also shopping for a treasured, classic, authentic American icon. In fact, shopping for vintage denim has become an extremely expensive, competitive, and lucrative business, especially on the Japanese market where fascination with American culture is almost a way of life. It's not unusual for a pair of Levi's from the 1950s to go for as much as $3,000.

So if what you're looking for is the real deal in vintage denim—jeans or jackets—a little history is required. According to denim experts, the fabric was first woven about A.D. 300 and supposedly used to make the sails of the Nina, Pinta, and Santa Maria. The popular cotton cloth was actu-

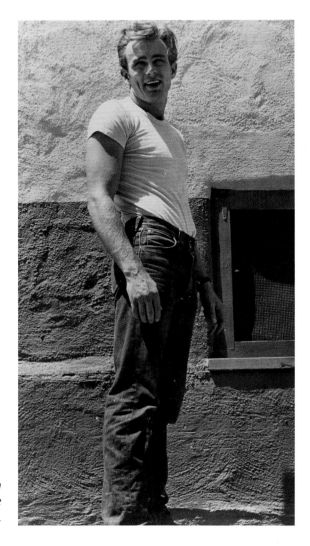

James Dean broke fashion barriers and launched an era as a rebellious and misunderstood youth in the 1955 film, Rebel Without a Cause.

1960: The word "overalls" is replaced by the word "jeans" in advertising.

1962: Styled jeans appear on Carnaby Street, London.

1963: Pre-shrunk Levi's are introduced.

1964: Jeans become part of the permanent collection at the Smithsonian Institution in Washington, D.C.

1965: Bell-bottomed jeans are patched and embroidered.

1966: Levi's airs its first television commercial.

Late 1970s: With the designer jean boom (Calvin Klein, Jordache, Gloria Vanderbilt, Bill Blass, Sergio Valente), the jeans industry manufactures 500,000 miles of jeans a year—enough to span the equator 20 times.

ally coined "denim" much later on. Nîmes, a town in the south of France known for manufacturing this particular fabric which was used primarily for upholstery purposes, takes the credit. The fabric was "de Nîmes" (from Nîmes), hence "denim." Sailors from Genoa, Italy, started wearing pants made from the sturdy, durable, and relatively lightweight cotton cloth. The sailors were called "genes" (being from Genoa), from which derived the word "jeans." The pant was also popular with sailors from the port of Dungri, India, hence the term "dungarees."

Although vintage Lee's and Wrangler's are hot items, Levi's seems to be the pièce de résistance among collectors, probably because Levi's were the first ones around. Lee jeans didn't come out until the late 1910s, and Wrangler entered the denim world in the late 1940s. Levi's on the other hand, started manufacturing denim "waist overalls" in the late 1800s, after Levi Strauss, a dry-goods business operator in San Francisco,

joined forces with Jacob Davis, who had invented the process to rivet the pocket corners on men's pants. And in 1890, the first pair of 501s, used to designate the copper-riveted overalls, was sold for about $1.25.

The appeal and versatility of denim goes without saying. Like chinos, jeans can be dressed up with a cashmere turtleneck or button-down shirt and blazer as easily as it can be dressed down with a T-shirt and a pair of sneakers.

and keep in mind...

- *Leather brand patches (instead of paper)*

- *Crotch rivet (discontinued in 1941)*

- *Buckle on the back of the jacket or pants (the first version of Levi's had these)*

- *Buttons instead of belt loops (to attach suspenders)*

- *Zinc buttons instead of copper (from 1938 to early 1950s)*

1978: Fiorucci launches tight, lie-on-the-floor-to-put-on jeans.

1979: Calvin Klein launches his jeans line with an adolescent Brooke Shields purring, "Nothing comes between me and my Calvins."

2001: The oldest known pair of Levi's in existence, found buried in mud in a Nevada mining town, is auctioned off on the Internet and sold for over $46,000. The 120-year-old pair is bought by the original manufacturers, Levi's Co. themselves.

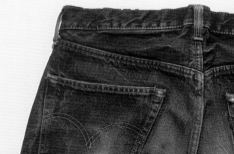

jeans' genes: what to look for in vintage levi's

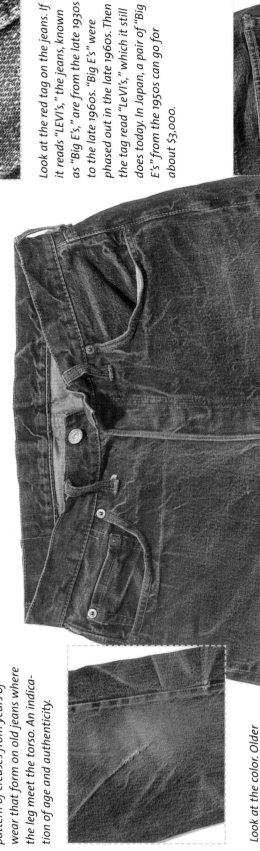

Look for "hige," a Japanese term for "whiskers," the cat-whisker-like pattern of creases from years of wear that form on old jeans where the leg meet the torso. An indication of age and authenticity.

Look at the red tag on the jeans. If it reads "LEVI's," the jeans, known as "Big E's," are from the late 1930s to the late 1960s. "Big E's" were phased out in the late 1960s. Then the tag read "LeVI's," which it still does today. In Japan, a pair of "Big E's" from the 1950s can go for about $3,000.

Look at the stitching on the back pockets. Single-stitching is older than double-stitching.

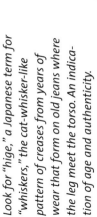

Look at the color. Older jeans tend to be darker. Indigo dye, a deep-purple blue dye used before the early 1970s, is highly desirable.

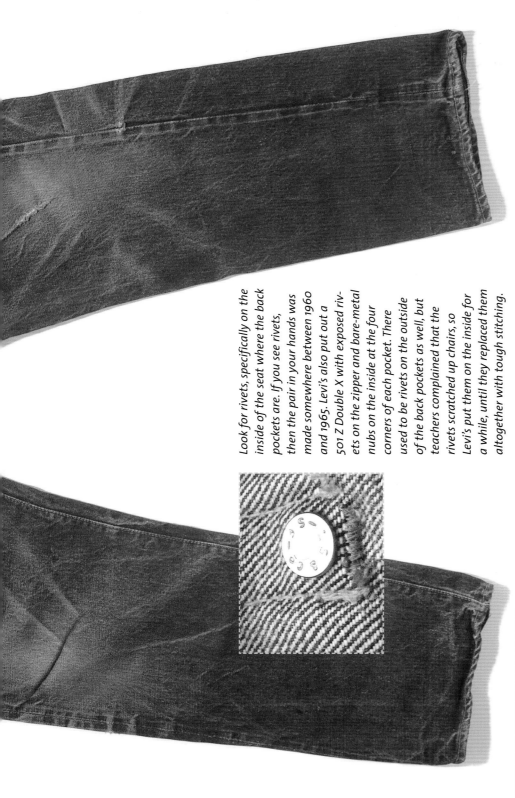

Look for rivets, specifically on the inside of the seat where the back pockets are. If you see rivets, then the pair in your hands was made somewhere between 1960 and 1965. Levi's also put out a 501 Z Double X with exposed rivets on the zipper and bare-metal nubs on the inside at the four corners of each pocket. There used to be rivets on the outside of the back pockets as well, but teachers complained that the rivets scratched up chairs, so Levi's put them on the inside for a while, until they replaced them altogether with tough stitching.

Turn the pair inside out. Check out whether the seam running down the leg has red thread woven through two white ones. Before 1971, Levi's used the end of the cloth bolt for the insides of their jeans and then in the early 1980s, it changed the way it dyed its jeans, which affected the color of the seams. These jeans are called "Red Lines," the trade name for 501s.

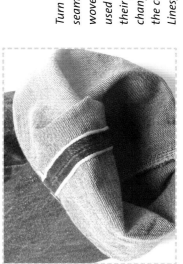

In the *Dictionary of American Slang*, jeans are described as "a pair of stiff, tight-fitting, tapered denim cowboy work pants, usually blue, with heavy reinforced seams and slash pockets."[110]

{western wear}

Western wear is a whole category in itself. The appeal of the new frontier and wide open spaces, the romantic vision of how the West was won, the promise of hope and unlimited horizons, starry-eyed romances with Roy Rogers, Annie Oakley, Davy Crockett, John Wayne, and Buffalo Bill, and the sheer nostalgia for classic Americana never goes out of style.

Western clothes have a unique style of their own. Some say that the classic American Western look "remains unchallenged as the epitome of virility in men's clothing." Derived from the cowboy's work clothes, "it is part national heritage and as such has made its way through twentieth-century

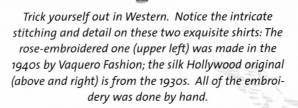

Trick yourself out in Western. Notice the intricate stitching and detail on these two exquisite shirts: The rose-embroidered one (upper left) was made in the 1940s by Vaquero Fashion; the silk Hollywood original (above and right) is from the 1930s. All of the embroidery was done by hand.

men's fashions…[It] gained enormous popularity in the thirties with the discovery that a visit to a dude ranch offered a splendid summer vacation."[11] They can be rough and rugged and right off the ranch: a checked cotton shirt or gabardine shirt with a checked yoke and cuffs, blue denim Levi's, a suede fringed jacket, a red bandana, and high-heeled black boots. Or fancy and flamboyant with rhinestones and embroidery: a bright red sateen shirt with sparkly accents, a rayon gabardine shirt with ornate embroidery and suede felt appliqués, or a Nudie-designed rhinestone-studded pair of hip-huggers. They can be fringed and worn with a pair of beat-up jeans (think John Voight in *Midnight*

SNAPS "Rodeo Ben" is credited for being the first to use snaps on Western shirts instead of buttons, as early as 1933. He came up with the idea after seeing a rodeo cowboy get snared when an opening in his button-front shirt got caught in the saddle's pummel. And unlike buttons, snaps don't get torn off during rough riding on the range. Some of the fanciest snaps are made of mother-of-pearl (debuting in the late 1940s), fancy turquoise inlays, or ocean pearl shank buttons.

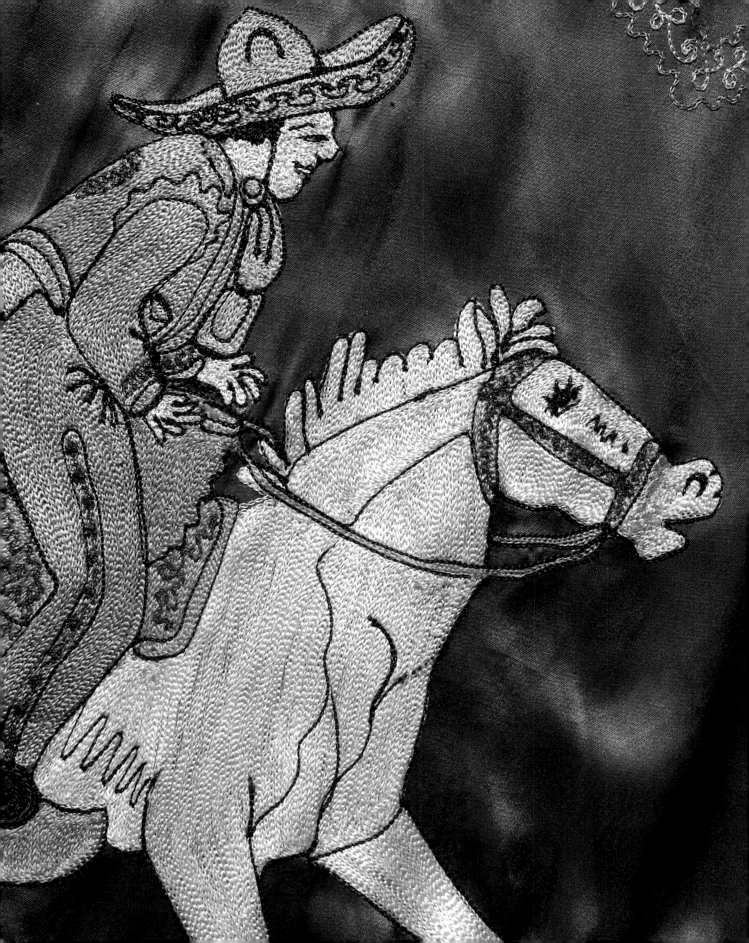

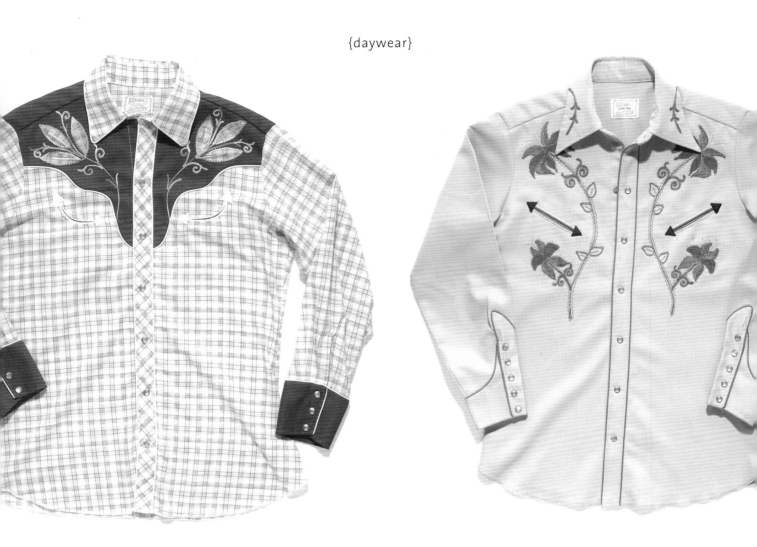

A pair of traditional H Bar C shirts feature embroidery, piped trim, crescent-shaped breast pockets. One has a dipped yoke, the other double-flat front pockets and Caballero cuffs.

western zest

In addition to the Western-style shirt and pants, the complete cowpuncher's dress includes a pair of black calf boots with patterned uppers, lizard boots, or pointy- or square-toed, Cuban-heeled cowboy boots; a black telescope-crown sombrero or a ten gallon hat by Stetson or Resistol; a Pendleton vest; a bandana or a heavyweight pure silk muffler with silver slip ring; suede or leather chaps; a leather, gator, or snake belt with fancy silver trim and buckle; hand-forged silver or steel spurs; and Silver, the horse.

Cowboy (1969) or John Travolta in *Urban Cowboy* (1980)) or gleaming with twenty-four carat gold lamé (think Elvis circa 1957) and fine detailing, piping, satin sheen, and flowing fringe (think Tammy Wynette, Patsy Cline, and Johnny Cash).

Western-style shirts were particularly popular in the 1950s, when "leisure wear" became a household name. Authentic styling with two-toned color combinations, open-neck lacing or pointed stitched yokes in front and back, dipped yokes, checkered patterns, piped trim, crescent-shaped chest pockets, double-flat front pockets, snaps (preferably mother-of-pearl), leather-trimmed sleeves, tapered cuffs, suede, felt, and leather appliqués, rhinestones, and embroidery were de rigueur. Cuffs vary from three snaps to what's called a five-snap Caballero (Spanish for "horse") cuff. Pocket styles include dart, saddlebag, flap, or two-point Arizona wing. Grab anything with an H–C label (pronounced H Bar C), considered the cream of the crop when it comes to designers and manufacturers of western-style shirts.

The authentic cowboy jean was first man-ufactured in the late 1940s. Blue Bell, a dungaree manufacturer in Philadelphia, collaborated with two men to design a pair of denims that would suit the needs and demands of cowboys on the ranch and in rodeos. One of them was a champion cowboy named Jim Shoulders, and the other was "Rodeo Ben" (a.k.a. Ben Lichtenstein), a tailor who specialized in making clothing for rodeo performers and cowboy movie stars. To endure life on the range, the jeans had to be every bit as durable as they were comfortable and practical. After lassoing professional cowboys and ranchers for their opinions and advice, a design was finally cut into the cloth. Blue Bell came up with a super-sturdy pair of jeans, complete with double-needle felled seams for durability, front pockets deep enough for gloves, back pockets reinforced to be tool-proof, flat copper rivets that won't rub the saddle, and a rise in the back high enough so that a man wouldn't have to sit on his billfold while in the saddle. The 13MWZ (which stands for 13 Variations, Men's Western Zipper) was born. The tongue-twisting name was changed to Wrangler, with a distinctive logo spelled out in rope-like lettering.

Be Western down to your toes with already-broken-in vintage cowboy boots.

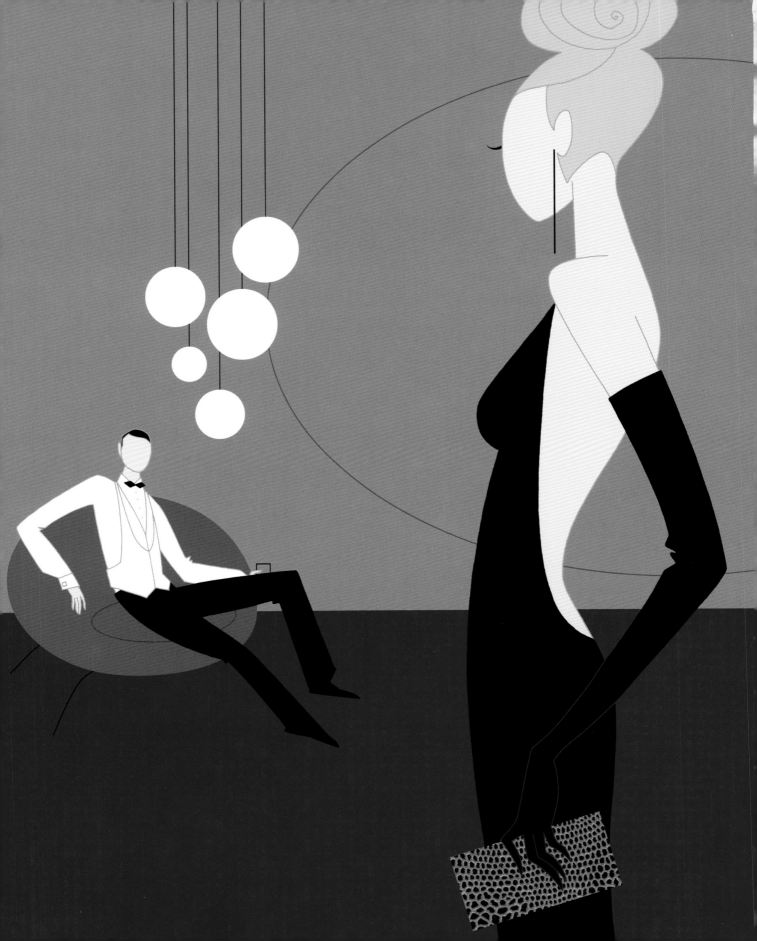

{4}

formalwear

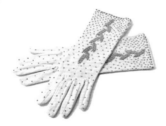

*"A dress makes no sense
unless it inspires men to want to take it off you."*

—Françoise Sagan

formally yours

The appeal of vintage formal wear lies in its diversity—there are at least six or seven different decades to chose from—in its quality, and, of course, in its price. Why blow a fortune on a contemporary designer look that'll be outdated by the time you get invited to your next formal, when you can invest in a fabulous, timeless piece that über-fashionistas can only dream of replicating?

The wonderful thing about vintage formalwear is that it's all out there. Bias-cut silks, velvets, and satins, and gentlemen's mourning coats from the 1920s and 1930s; embroidery and bugle-bead-accentuated crepes and jerseys from the late 1940s and early 1950s; full-skirted dresses and wood grain moiré tuxedos from the 1950s; empire cocktail dresses, Jackie O sheaths, and men's psychedelic evening jackets from the 1960s; mint-colored ruffled tuxedo shirts and

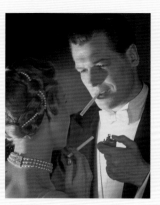

Rekindle the elegance of the past in a vintage tux and watch the sparks fly!

Victorian-inspired dresses from the 1970s. True, some of the heavenly fabrics used to create yesteryear's eveningwear—beaded and sequined satins, ultra-delicate laces and chiffons, sumptuously hand-painted silks—tend to be more fragile, so the likelihood of some damage is a reality. A spill of Champagne or a smidgen of lipstick here, maybe a cigarette burn or a passionate heat-of-the-moment tear there, anything's possible. On the other hand, eveningwear has always been reserved for special occasions; so by definition, it's exempted from daily wear-and-tear. If the piece was properly cleaned and stored, even forty or fifty years ago, it's probably outlasted its daywear counterparts, sliding elegantly and unscathed into a new generation of wardrobes. And chances are, if you're going to find a gem in the world of vintage, it's hiding in the formalwear aisle.

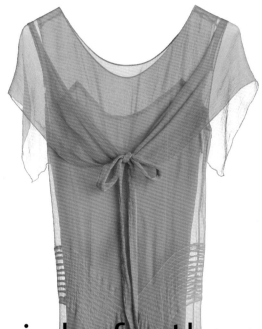

"Formalwear is by far the most popular section for vintage shoppers."

The sheer elegance of this bias-cut silk chiffon gown from the thirties will outshine every other dress in the room.

{women's formalwear}

"There's something inexplicably romantic about wearing a dress that someone maybe two or three generations ago wore on a happy occasion, and of giving it renewed life under similar circumstances."

Vintage eveningwear pieces for women are some of the most desirable items on today's market. The reason is simple. Whether it's the soft, elegant, romantic silk satins and chiffons from the twenties, mermaid-style dresses from the thirties, lavish dinner gowns from the forties and fifties, or straight, simple shifts from the sixties, the cuts are marvelous, the fabrics superb, and the colors splendid. And it's amazing how contemporary these garments look.

Hollywood has recently discovered the appeal of vintage eveningwear. Celebrities, for whom purchasing the latest couture piece is not a financial burden, have instead opted for anything but contemporary duds. The likes of Nicole Kidman, Julia Roberts, Marcia Gay Harden, Meg Ryan, Courteney Cox Arquette, Renée Zellweger, Lisa Kudrow, and Winona Ryder have been making dramatic entrances at formal events in sophisticated "hand-me-downs." Wearing vintage, they claim, provides an elegance, quality, and comfort they admire. Marcia Gay Harden, the 2001 Academy Award winner for her role in *Pollock*, admits loving vintage because "it's a means of reinvention—and an actress is reinventing things all the time—whether she's in or out of character."[12]

More important, though, it provides the priceless assurance that no one else in the room will be seen wearing the same outfit.

Looking every bit the 1940s glamour girl in her strapless red satin gown at the 2001 Academy Awards, Harden explains that vintage formalwear "...is like a habit, it lures you in. First you discover one decade, then another, then another."[13] She is not the only one lured.

Winona Ryder struts her stuff in a vintage Edward Sabesta gown at the 1994 Academy Awards.

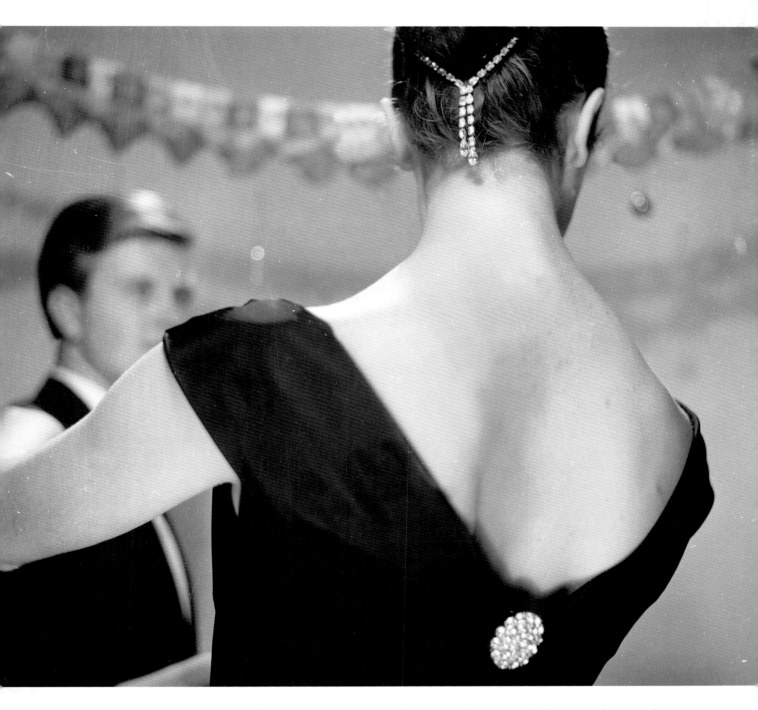

In the 1950s, dramatic backless dresses, strapless gowns, and low-cut necklines epitomized post-war luxury and femininity, and a bare back is still an attention-grabber. Lavish costume jewelry enhances the glamour.

Demi Moore wowed the 1992 Oscar crowd in her forties lavender-gray halter gown. Winona Ryder turned heads in her late-fifties Edward Sabesta white beaded and fringed dress at the 1994 Academy Awards, and with her 1940s Pauline Trigère cream satin-lined gown at Oscars 2000. At the 1995 Academy Awards, Diane Keaton was stunning in a fifties black suit with diamond-shaped cutout jacket. At Oscars 2001, Renée Zellweger simply glowed in her 1960s strapless canary yellow Jean Desses chiffon gown, and Julia Roberts picked up her award in a vintage Valentino. And at an April 2001 screening of her film *Moulin Rouge*, Nicole Kidman seduced in a slinky late-'70s satin fringed gown by Loris Azzaro.

But of course a vintage gown does not have to be couture or carry a designer label to be exquisite. Style, quality, and attention to detail seem to remain consistent and of high standard in vintage formalwear, regardless of the designer or manufacturer. What makes many of these gowns so priceless and original is that they are not in fashion, but above it. A pale lavender chiffon beaded cocktail dress from the twenties; a thirties dress with a dramatic neckline featuring wide, scalloped edges or a ruffled collar; a 1940s luscious velvet evening gown with a broad neckline and sweeping skirt; a gold moiré gown with a square neck and short sleeves from the same era; a bustle-back taffeta evening gown with a round neck, ruched sleeves, and an attached crinoline from the fifties; a black halter tulle dress with rhinestone trim, also from the fifties; or a shimmering red cocktail dress with matching short jacket accentuated with beads and gold buttons from the sixties…these are just a few examples of the glorious "no-name" options available for under $200, a mere fraction of what a new gown, most likely of lesser quality and inferior style, would cost today!

Make your vintage gown stand out even more by adding a modern twist: Wear a pair of fabulous spiked heels, wrap yourself in a luxurious pashmina shawl, and hide all your necessaries in a precious rhinestone-studded clutch purse. One word of advice, though: it's best to avoid going head-to-toe vintage, unless you want to look like an extra in *Titanic*.

DESIGNER PROFILE:

Pauline Trigère

Unlike other designers who sketch their creations before cutting them into cloth, fashion doyenne Pauline Trigère's creative juices run through her scissors. With Zorro-like flair and precision, she slashes directly into fabric draped on live models, yielding impeccably cut clothes that blend elegance with practicality. Born in France, Trigère fled Hitler's troops in 1937 and came to live in the United States with her husband, mother, and two sons. After separating from her husband, she needed to find a way to support herself and her children, and found work as an assistant to Manhattan designer Hattie Carnegie.

By 1942, Trigère had started her own collection with eleven dresses, which quickly got the attention of several key department stores. In 1949, she won the first of three prestigious American Fashion Critics' Coty Awards, and in 1961 caused shockwaves up and down Seventh Avenue when she hired Beverly Valdes, the first African-American runway model to work a major show. Trigère was also one of the first designers to introduce less traditional fabrics, like wool and cotton, into eveningwear. Her signature styles include reversible capes and jumpsuits. Her remarkable gowns from the forties and fifties have caught the eye of Winona Ryder and Julianna Margulies.

This gorgeous Pauline Trigère, made of printed chiffon, is a perfect example of the fluidity and elegance inherent in the designer's pieces.

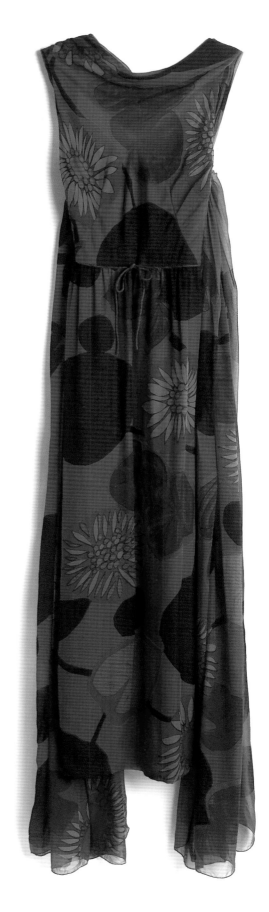

{gowns}

Formalwear is by far the most popular section among vintage shoppers. The reason is simple. When women go out to buy something formal, chances are they're buying it with a specific event in mind. And if you have an eventful calendar in front of you, filled with glittery formal events, that can mean a lot of different outfits to buy. As we all know, wearing the same dress at back-to-back parties is not even a remote possibility, especially if the ex-boyfriend and his new squeeze happen to be on the guest list as well. And we've all done the mental math at the register: "You mean for the price of this slinky number (o.k., it's cute but there's really not that much fabric to it…just a couple of spaghetti straps…), I could have gotten two pairs of pants, that sweater that I've been dying for, some sexy lingerie, those awesome leather boots that what's-her-face has, and a manicure?!?"

Well, this is where vintage formalwear really saves the day. We're talking savings in the hundreds, possibly thousands. But let's be clear on something: that Pauline Trigère on Winona, albeit vintage, probably cost her a pretty penny, even if it was "used." The truth is that because vintage formalwear has become so hot, vintage haute couture—Chanel, Saint Laurent, Valentino, de la Renta, Jacques Fath, Christian Dior, Guy Laroche, Norman Norell, Halston, Balenciaga, Carven, to name just a few—costs a pretty penny, no matter how "used" it is. It's not unheard of for a 1950s Balenciaga to go for $1,200, for example, or for a 1950s silk brocade Christian Dior evening dress to go for $1,500. Where vintage formalwear comes through, however, is with those smaller, independent designers whose names have not (yet) been discovered, but

Above: A sweet silk chiffon dress from the fifties with a tulle overlay. Right: an off-the-shoulder chiffon gown from the forties with exquisite detail. See the close-up on page 122 showing its beautiful fabric-covered buttons.

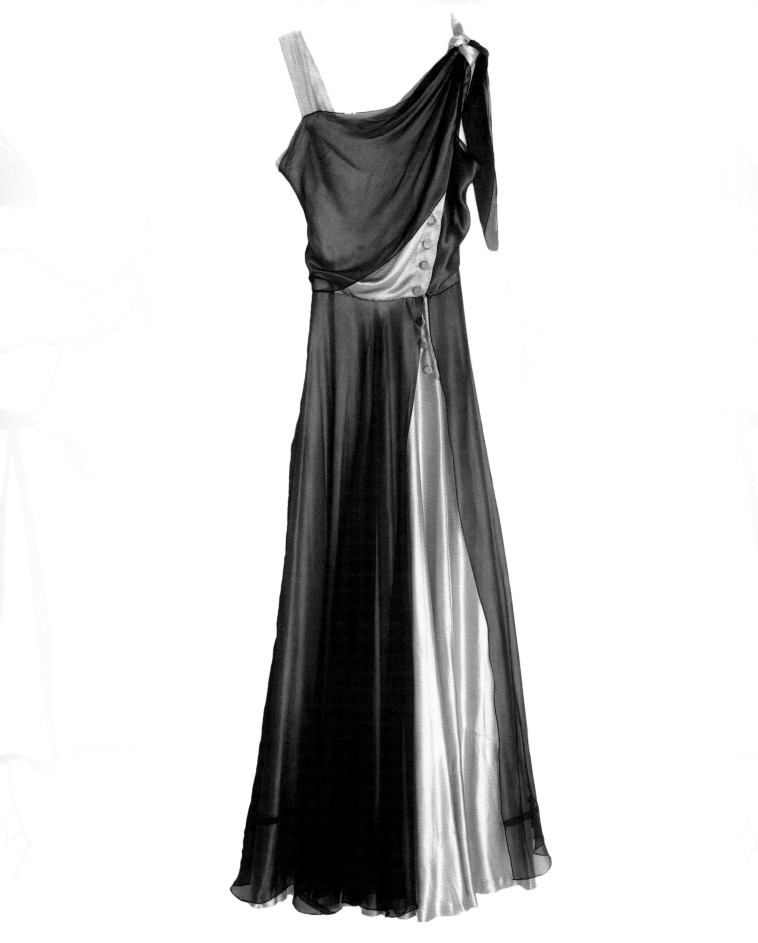

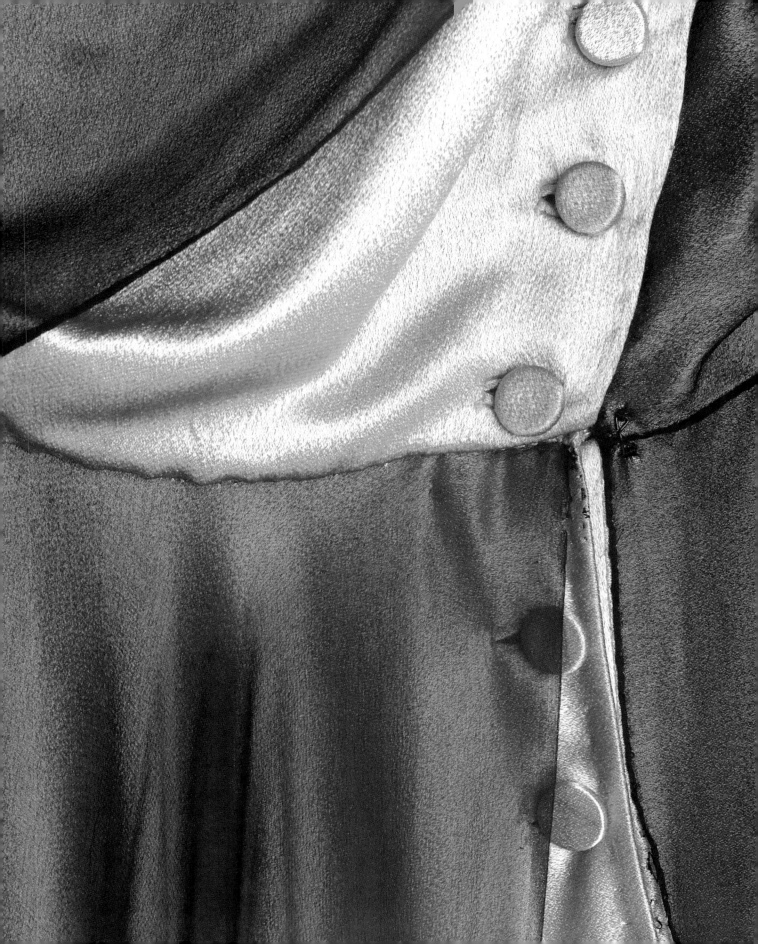

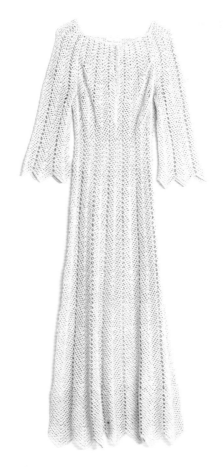

A silver crochet metallic dress from the late sixties.

whose dresses and gowns are often as sumptuous in quality and look as some of the big guns'. That's because many women who could not afford to buy couture had pieces copied by their seamstress. Although the design was technically no longer an "original," the workmanship was often as extensive—hand-stitched hems and hand-finished trim—and the quality of the fabric as good. And remember, don't judge a book by its cover, or in this case, a dress by its (lack of) label. Just because something is missing a label doesn't mean it should be passed over. In fact, it was not uncommon for women who bought their clothes overseas to cut out all labels before passing back through customs upon their return to the U.S. Naughty for them—lucky for you!

When you're shopping for eveningwear, keep in mind what suits your particular body type. In the thirties, for example, sleek, and slinky "column" or "pillar gowns" were cut on the bias, Hollywood style. Although these figure-hugging beauties are undeniably sexy, especially in rich, clingy fabrics like satin and silk, they're unfortunately not for everyone. Merciless in that they can reveal even the tiniest of flaws, thirties' gowns are best reserved for those who have the genes of a silver-screen diva.

If, like the average woman, you have several strategically placed curves here and there (maybe you are a bit heavier below the waist than above?), then dresses from the early 1950s might be more your cup of tea. Fifties dresses, designed to emphasize the hourglass figure, feature tight-fitting bodices topping skirts that flair out over endless layers of crinoline. As you can imagine, these tend to flatter virtually any body type. The fullness of the skirt is beautifully offset by the display of a little skin—thanks to plunging necklines, back cleavage, bare shoulders, or off-the-shoulder bodices that can be complemented by vintage costume jewelry. Satin and silk wraps, fur stoles, and velvet boleros wrap up the look in style.

Towards the end of the decade and certainly into the next, waistless shifts and sheaths detracted attention from the torso, drawing it down towards the leg, sometimes climbing up to the upper thigh, causing quite a sensation. Flowing chiffon dresses that looked as if they had their bottom halves chopped off dominated the late-night social scene. If your lower body is indeed your best feature, this might be the style to go with.

Although the seventies have more than once been referred to as "the decade that taste forgot," some of the most classic and enduringly stylish evening gowns have emerged from that era. Above all, one particular designer's influence created ripple effects throughout the industry. Halston's play with flowing jersey and ultrasuede made for graceful shapes that sensually followed the body's lines without overpowering them with structure. The dresses naturally and comfortably enhanced what was already there, in a sexy yet discreet way.

In contrast to this simple elegance, the seventies were also responsible for "big" dresses, over-the-top gowns with lots of flowing fabric, layers of exotic textures and graphic designs, unusual textiles, uneven hemlines, Indian prints, large sleeves, beads and pearls, stitching, and waist sashes. Think the Mamas and the Papas or Stevie Nicks. Designers like British-born Zandra Rhodes made waves with her "big dress"

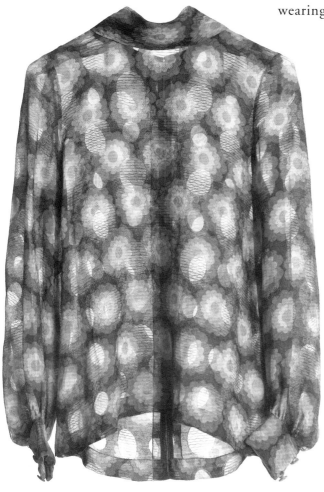

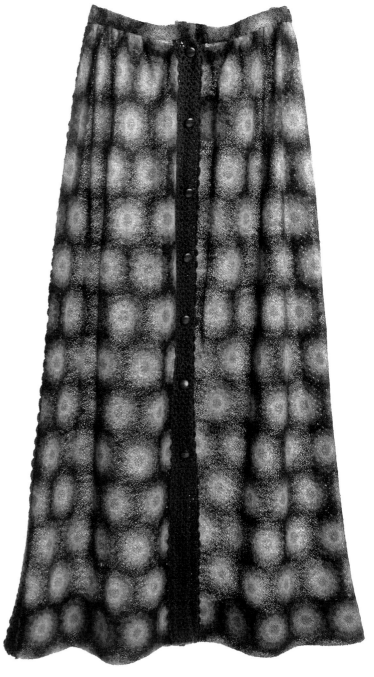

A Christian Dior 1960s original.

creations, fashioning pieces with two sets of armholes (one cut just above the waist), for example, or with seams sewn on the outside and hems lopped off with shears. If you're fortunate enough to come across one of these during a vintage expedition, don't worry about your body type—just snatch it up fast. Such works of art always make great conversation pieces, and can sometimes be modified or altered without compromising the original intent of the the designer.

{wedding dresses}

Women who are looking for a dress for the "Big Day" are turning to vintage for something special in which to walk down the aisle. Particularly with vintage wedding dresses, history, sentimentality, and tradition play an important role. There's something inexplicably romantic about wearing a dress that someone maybe two or three generations ago wore on a happy occasion, and of giving it renewed life under similar circumstances. Intricate detailing, delicate beadwork, high-quality fabrics such as satin, silk organza, and chantilly lace (which is rarely used anymore but photographs regally), silk ribbon embroidery, three or four layers of chiffon, boning and built-in corsets, extra trim, pearl work, and hand-appliquéd flowers are just a few reasons why vintage is so desirable for that most important of dresses. That kind of craftsmanship would be cost-prohibitive today.

The vintage wedding gown you pick out will likely be in excellent shape, since it's probably been worn only once. At most, it'll need a bit of tailoring here and there; but any wedding dress—new or old—needs to be fitted. Don't pay too close attention to size. Because of diet, lifestyle, and exercise, modern-day brides tend to be larger than women of generations past, especially in the rib cage and shoulders. The average size of a vintage dress is a 4, compared to today's 14. Waists were fashionably tiny from the '40s through the late '60s. Women invested in waist-reducing foundation garments like corsets, girdles, and boned bodices. But fortunately, tailors often had the foresight to know that figures expand and dresses are often passed down, so seams and hems were more generous, sometimes with up to three or four inches to spare. Extra fabric in the train might also be used to enlarge portions of the bodice, if need be. Whatever money you save on the dress, you can apply toward the honeymoon. Or a case of vintage wine.

A selection of vintage wedding gowns might include the following: a 1920s belted chemise

Right: A glimpse of the blushing bride, Shirley Jones, in a princess wedding dress with sweetheart neckline, fitted body, and ballerina skirt, just before marrying Jack Cassidy in 1956.

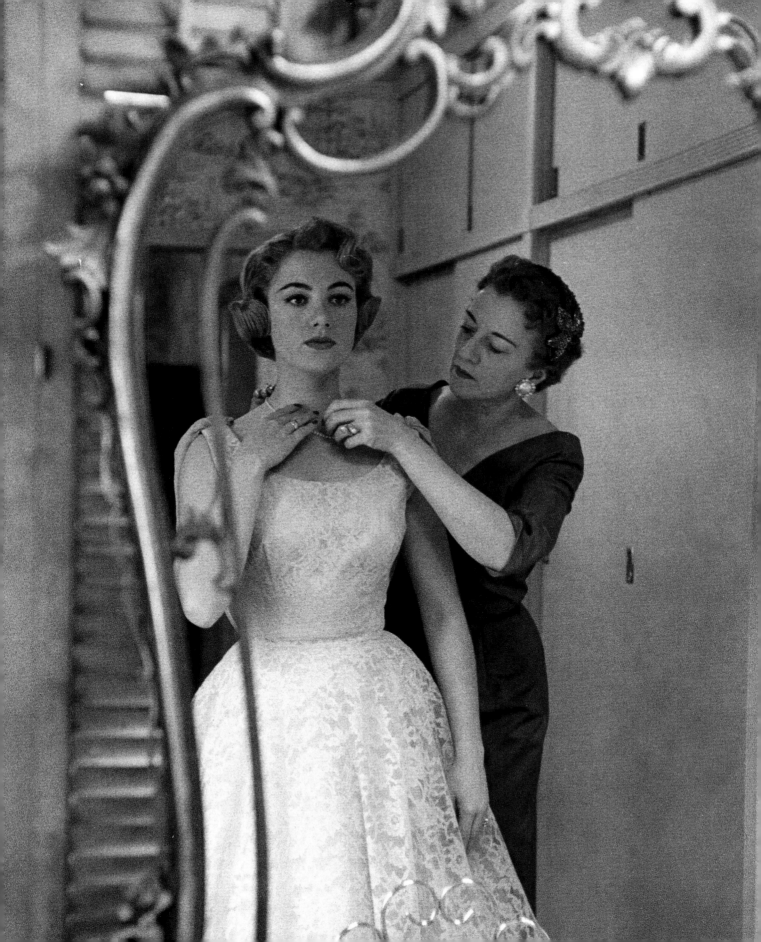

{men's formalwear}

"There's not a single woman out there who wouldn't swoon if she saw a man in trim-cut pants with an evening tailcoat from the 1920s."

Okay, so you never thought you'd see the day when '70s powder-blue ruffled tuxedo shirts would once again rule the dance floor. Or when Johnny Carson's tapered pants from the '60s would inspire what's trotting down the runways. But in today's parlance, "they're baaaack!"

Like women, an increasing number of men—David Arquette, Chris Isaak, and Johnny Depp, just to name a few—have been going the vintage route, especially for formalwear. Classic mourning coats and piqued waistcoats with soft-roll lapels from the 1920s, postboy waistcoats from the late 1930s, wood grain moiré and taffeta tuxedos in riots of colors and prints from the 1950s, lean and modern 1950s sack suits popularized by Brooks Brothers and J. Press, and stand-up collars from the 1930s, all of these are being resurrected and worn enthusiastically by men with style. Eager to step out of the cookie-cutter tuxedo mold that plagues contemporary designers, men are opting for an elegance of yesteryear that outstrips anything off today's racks.

thirties side orders

Must-have accessories for a night on the town include a black or white butterfly tie of moderate width; plain white or black pearl studs; black silk socks or hose; silk underwear; plain crystal shirt studs; a red carnation; a diamond and platinum dress pocket watch and chain; black patent leather shoes, highly polished Russian-calf low evening shoes, or opera pumps; a tall silk or ribbed silk collapsible or crushable opera hat; a white silk crepe scarf with fringed ends, or a knitted muffler loosely draped around the neck; a black overcoat; white kid gloves; a fouet (a gadget designed to eliminate bubbles from champagne); and Lauren Bacall.

An elegant six-button wool vest, shirt, and tie from the 1930s.
Opposite: Cab Calloway put the zoot suit on the map in the 1943 film, Stormy Weather.

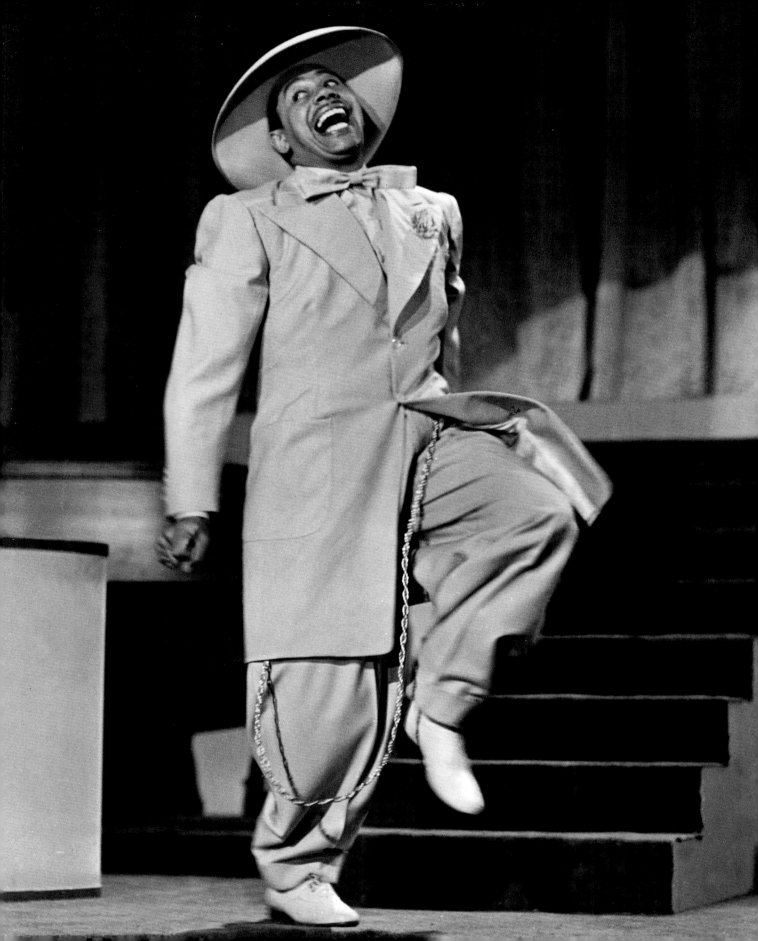

{tails, tuxes, & dinner jackets}

There is not a single woman out there who wouldn't swoon if she saw a man in trim-cut pants with an evening tailcoat from the 1920s, complete with satin-faced lapels, bone buttons, a wing collar, a simple large white pearl in the shirt, cuff-links to match, and patent-leather low cut boots. Or one sporting a dinner jacket with rounded notched lapels, a wing collar, a butterfly bowtie, and a white, double-breasted evening waistcoat with an oval opening.

The popular single-breasted dinner jackets from the twenties made way for less formal double-breasted ones in the thirties, a style favored by Palm Beach-goers and kings alike (King Alfonso XIII of Spain was partial to them). The double-breaster was cut in two different styles: the English version with high-placed buttons (either the lower or the top button is to be buttoned, but not both) with its wide lap, which means that only a small area of the shirt front was visible; and the American two-button version (only the lower button was to be buttoned), with a narrower lap thus exposing more of the shirt's front.

The early forties exhibited a preference for double-breasted midnight blue dinner jackets with four brass buttons and black satin shawl lapels, worn with trousers draped ever so slightly over low-cut patent leather evening shoes, or single-breasted shawl-collar white jackets worn with midnight blue pants with a single braid down the side and a midnight blue cummerbund. But with the onset on World War II restrictions, only the single-breasted dinner jacket remained, of which a midnight blue version with narrow shawl collar, straight lines, and narrow shoulders seeped its way into the fifties. The more conservative and cautious climate of the early fifties also saw an uncanny concern and

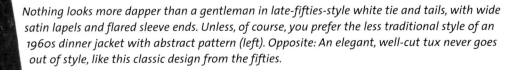

Nothing looks more dapper than a gentleman in late-fifties-style white tie and tails, with wide satin lapels and flared sleeve ends. Unless, of course, you prefer the less traditional style of an 1960s dinner jacket with abstract pattern (left). Opposite: An elegant, well-cut tux never goes out of style, like this classic design from the fifties.

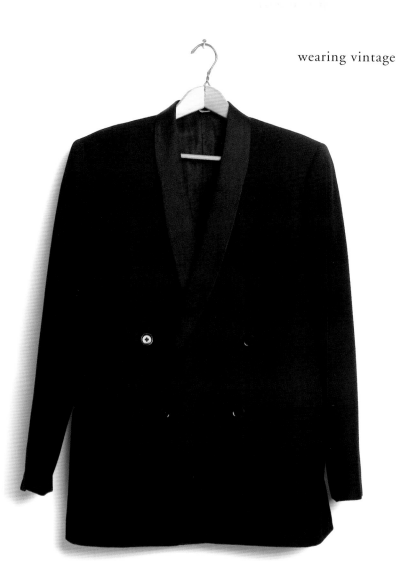

waist not *During the beginning of the twentieth century, the waistcoat was double-breasted, usually white piqué or linen with a deep rolled collar or single-breasted with short rounded points, a rolled collar and five buttons. A backless model with only a strap and buckle at the waistline was introduced in the early twenties. It was usually single-breasted with a V opening and three buttons, and it was considered more comfortable than one with a back. The postboy, popularized in the thirties, was made of flannel or box cloth and had lapels and flaps on its pockets. For some reason, yellow was a popular color. The cummerbund, a broad silk sash that sometimes had horizontal pleats, gained popularity in the late twenties. It was often worn instead of a waistcoat on warm evenings. Popular cummerbund colors in the forties were black, midnight blue, bright red, or maroon, quite a contrast from the parfait colors of the fifties (blueberry, orange, strawberry, and raspberry) and the paisley and snowflake patterns of the seventies.*

'40s and '50s
dos and don'ts

"Don't shove the opera hat to open—just tap the brim on your palm. To close the topper, press the crown against your chest, but never close it unless necessary for packing.

Trousers with tail coat always carry double braid and break over instep.

For hose you may wear lightweight black wool as correctly as silk. Take your choice.

The starched shirt should have a white pique bosom. The cuffs are single and extend slightly beyond the jacket sleeve. Wear a bold wing collar.

The bow tie, of course, should be of white pique and it can match your shirt bosom and waistcoat. And it's easy to tie, so wear it that way.

The gloves should be of spotless white kid, mocha, or chamois. Chamois, you know, is washable, and the others are readily cleaned. They all last for years.

The pleated cummerbund in black, midnight blue, or maroon silk may be substituted for a black, midnight blue, or white waist-coat with the evening jacket; either the midnight blue or white being accepted for resort wear.

The backless waistcoats, tailored in white piqué, black, or mid-night blue silk, has become an established fashion simply because the absence of extra fabric in back makes it much more comfortable than those with backs. Always wear the waistcoat snugly and be sure your starched shirt front is short enough so that it doesn't dive into the tops of your trousers or extend at the sides under your suspenders." [14]

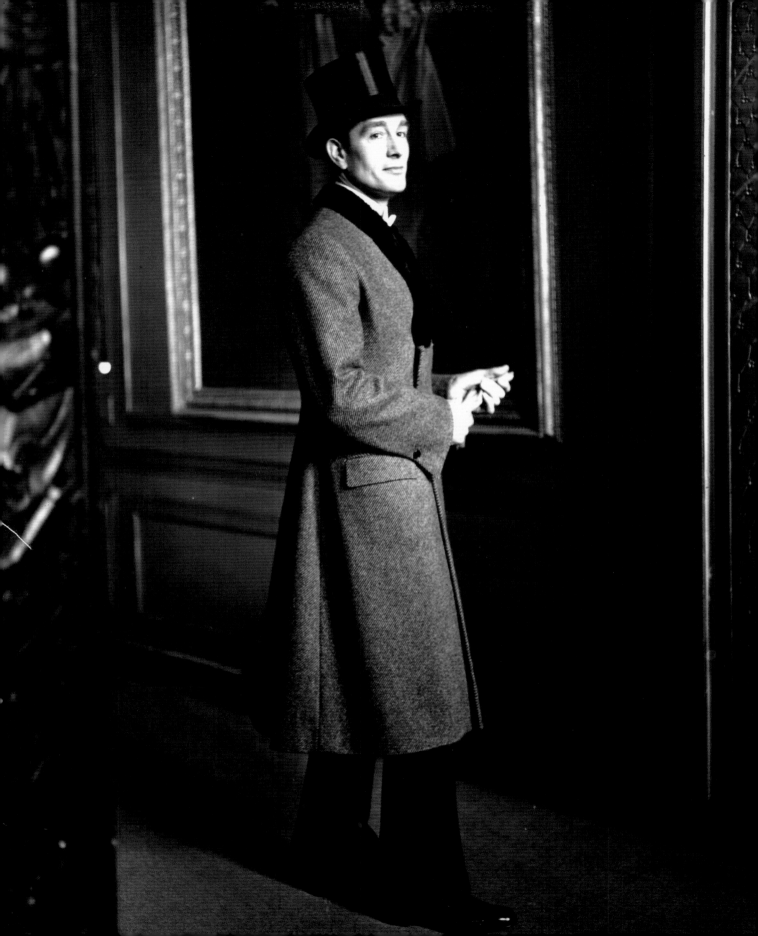

awareness for the etiquette of formal dressing.

In mid decade, though, things began to relax a bit, something that was reflected in fresh parfait colors such as strawberry, orange sherbert, raspberry, lime, lemon, or powder blue. The color scheme continued throughout the fifties, when bright red and bold tartan dinner jackets became popular. But the "Continental Look" dinner jacket, with peaked lapels and satin piping and braid, marked a new period of evening elegance. In black or silver gray mohair, it inspired a whole breed of richer evening accessories like cummerbunds with honeycomb designs, dress shirts with fine tucked pleats, and fancy bow ties.

The "Regency Look" of the sixties, however, quickly gained popularity. The "Regency Look" was a lightly padded double-breasted dinner jacket that flared to the skirt, with two sets of buttons, wide lapels, a small cutaway front exposing little of the shirt, and pronounced side or center vents, worn with plain-front trousers.

The trim, high-fashion silhouette, is ideally suited for a tall man with a fit physique.

The Nehru jacket made its first appearance in the United States in the mid sixties. The brocade or velvet jacket was inspired by the garment favored by Indian Prime Minister Jawaharlal Nehru. Worn with a white turtleneck, it remains an original approach to eveningwear, and it's a total knock-out. Toward the close of the decade, classic dinner white was back in style. With flapped pockets, flaring, peaked lapels, and white satin lining, the coat looks stunning with a white dinner shirt, white bow tie, and piped black or white pants.

The seventies startled and sparkled with color and permissiveness. Silk dinner jackets in lemon-lime and cream with contrasting colored shirts, ruffled dress shirts in red and blue check (yikes!), and paisley cummerbunds tossed the penguin look right out the window. Topped with a satin-lined black opera cape, opting for the '70s vintage formalwear look is certainly a way to leave your mark.

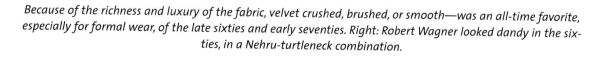

Because of the richness and luxury of the fabric, velvet crushed, brushed, or smooth—was an all-time favorite, especially for formal wear, of the late sixties and early seventies. Right: Robert Wagner looked dandy in the sixties, in a Nehru-turtleneck combination.

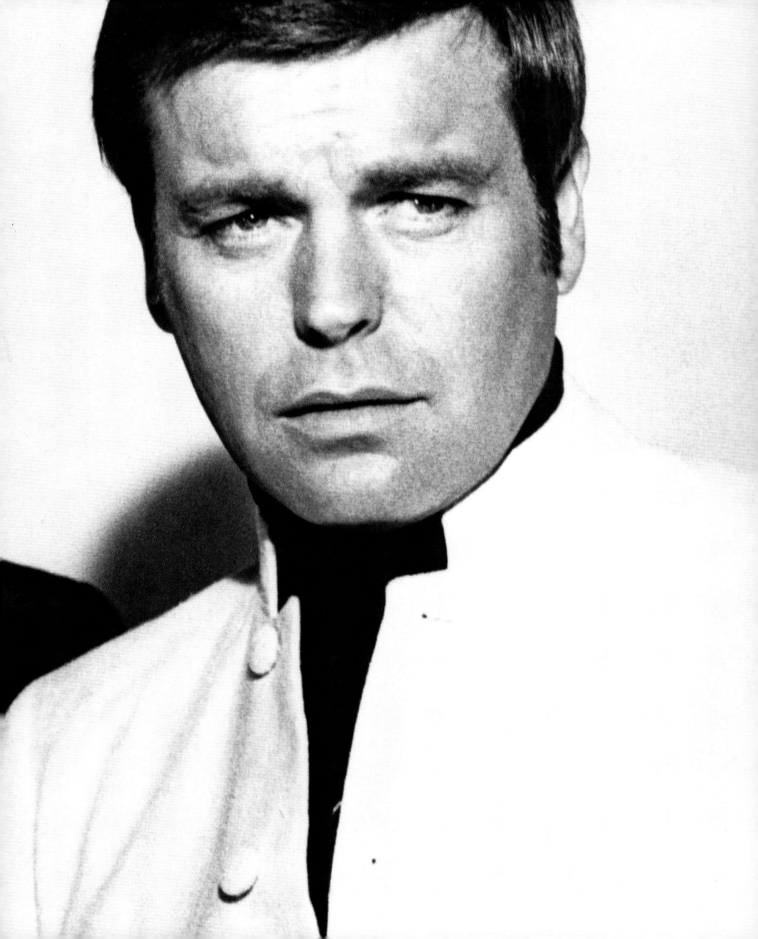

{suits}

Whatever your stature, taste, and style, there's a perfect vintage suit out there, practically tailored for you. From the Zoot, the extreme exaggeration of the suit from the early forties to the broad-shouldered and extended lapel "bold look" of the same decade, to the short "Continental" jacket with shaped waistline from the fifties or the polyester-knit suit of the seventies, eveningwear options and alternatives to a tux or tails abound.

If what tickles your fancy is the long, lean look, the "natural-shoulder suit" popular in the twenties is right up your alley. With straight-hanging lines and short, narrow lapels (sometimes the lapels are no wider than 2$\frac{1}{3}$ inches), the favored model is the simple single-breasted version, with a three- or four-button front. Worn with pants cuffed to a 17 or 18-

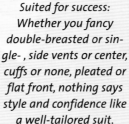

Suited for success: Whether you fancy double-breasted or single-, side vents or center, cuffs or none, pleated or flat front, nothing says style and confidence like a well-tailored suit.

inch width, the suit is primarily available in such austere colors as medium gray, brown, navy blue, with an occasional splash of tan, or blue gray. The lighter-shaded suit was also dubbed the "ice cream suit" because it also came in a husky diagonal tweed fabric, reminiscent of a waffle-like cone.

The perfect foundation garment for your summer wardrobe is, without a doubt, the double-breasted or three-button single-breasted tan gabardine suit, popularized in the thirties. Unlike the heavier wools and tweeds that are notorious for giving twenties' suits their masculine shape and almost stiff look, suits in the thirties were made of lighter-weight fabrics such as seersucker, tropical worsted, Palm Beach cloth, and linen, and are cut in a more relaxed shape. Jackets have broader shoulders and

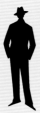

rules and regs *The War Production Board regulations had a tremendous impact on men's—and women's—fashions. The first area it affected was all suits containing wool. Two-trouser suits, cutaway coats, double-breasted dinner jackets, patch pockets, back, side, and front pleats, tucks, yokes, flaps, and cuffs were all eliminated. Jackets and pants were made shorter and narrower, creating a streamlined suit with no frills or fancy extras.*

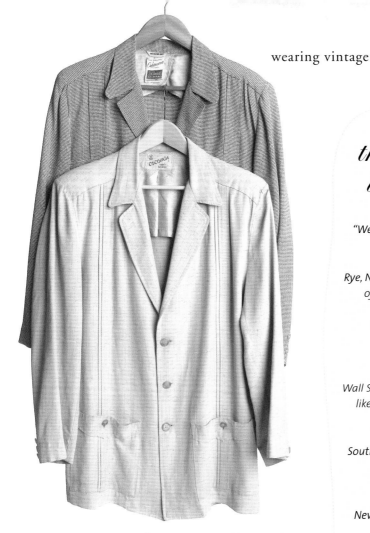

Late 1940s resort jackets were pressed into service as semi-formalwear in tropical climes.

waists are nipped in at the front and sides; trousers are high-waisted, double-pleated, and full cut.

By the mid to late thirties, suits with extra fullness in the chest and over the shoulder blades for added freedom of movement and the sake of comfort and ease made their way into the closet of every man of style. The drape suit, also known as the "British blade," the "British lounge," or

the most prominent birthplaces of style

"*Westbury, Long Island: Where the polo-playing set spend a great deal of time.*

Rye, New York: Where the Biltmore Country Club is one of the most important style centers in the U.S.

New York Stock Exchange: The birthplace of New York business style.

Yale: The undergraduate, often with a Wall Street career in his future, already acts and dresses like the young broker type who haunts New York's financial district.

Southampton, Long Island: The watering place where sands are made of platinum and the waters of sapphire.

Newport, Rhode Island: Has a decidedly high social caste that originated with the 400 in the Gay Nineties and has lasted down through the thrilling thirties.

Park Avenue: Where young brokers live and play, in the after-dark twin of Wall Street.

Palm Beach, Florida: To try to express the fashion significance of Palm Beach is like trying to explain the beauty of a woman.

Princeton: Where a large portion of the student body are some of the top-rankers in American social, financial, and diplomatic circles. They spend their vacations abroad and in general reflect the younger generation's version of what is being done in the smart world of their elders."[15]

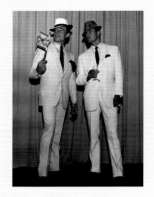

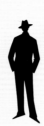

the white suit *The white suit has always been a romantic alternative in the world of fashion. While always lurking in the South as a viable option (something Rhett Butler seduced Scarlett O'Hara with, or F. Scott Fitzgerald's Jay Gatsby showed up in at garden parties), the white suit—especially in linen—remains a spotless classic. Paired with a silver shirt and a gold-colored tie, white doeskin bucks and a gold pocket watch, it is irresistible.*

the "lounge suit," first appeared in sharkskin, then in flannel, tweed, and saxony. The casual, elegant suit was favored in blue, gray, and blue-gray, but had a huge following in colorful plaids with wide peaked lapels, cuffed sleeves and two highly placed buttons. But at the beginning of the next decade, with an imminent world war, the suit became less colorful and more conservative. Gray flannel and dark blue with chalk pinstripes conformed to the fabric-conserving regulations of the War Production Board. Cuffs, pleats, and overlapping waistbands were immediately eliminated, yielding a taller, slimmer physique, ideal for today's athletic builds.

Despite the lean years surrounding World War II, there is one suit that managed to sneak its way into popularity—albeit discreetly—which is a very popular one among vintage shoppers. The Zoot suit, which made its first appearance in a store in Gainesville, Georgia, in 1939, is an extreme exaggeration of a suit. With padded,

boxy shoulders and a tapered waist, its hemline reaching almost to the knees, the Zoot suit jacket had slash pockets and pegged sleeves, and was worn with pleated, wide-legged trousers. Made popular by band-leader Cab Calloway, the suit quickly earned the nickname "the badge of the hoodlums," as it was a favorite among "hep" and gangster crowds of the day. Eventually banned by the War Production Board, it has now emerged as a favorite among contemporary swing dancers, due in part to its comfort and high style.

As a reaction to the austerity and turmoil of the war years, the "bold look" showed self-confidence and assurance, guaranteeing stature and presence. With broad and padded shoulders, wide lapels that were cut longer to accentuate height, lower-set buttons (think Gary Cooper and Cary Grant), the suit was heavily accessorized: it was worn with a widespread "command" or spread collar shirt with big buttons, a Windsor-knotted tie, a pocket handkerchief, thick-soled blucher shoes, heavy cuff links, wide tie clasps, and a snap-brim hat. New man-made fibers resulted in revolutionary fabric blends such as "doeskin," with the feel of cashmere but stronger than wool. A rainbow of colors was also introduced to men's suits, with browns, blues, tans, greens, and grays the prominent forerunners. With post-war détente leading into the more conservative climate of the late forties and fifties, the bold look gave way to a more cautious approach to fashion. A new, trim effect with a trend away from broad shoulders yielded

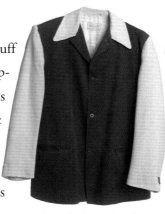

A three-button, two-tone gabardine and tweed blazer from the forties, made by Hollywood Sportswear Co. offers a casual alternative to a traditional suit jacket.

straight-hanging lines, short jackets with minimal padding, narrow lapels and trousers (dare we even say that they fit snugly?) blew into town with the cold war. The "sack suit," in a sea of olive drab and charcoal gray, was made popular by Brooks Brothers and J. Press. It had natural shoulders with a thin silhouette and thin lapels, and was described by many as sleek, elongating (by closing the top two buttons of the jacket, the wearer looked even lankier), slenderizing, forgiving, nondescript, and almost shapeless. (Think Rock Hudson, Tony Randall, and Gregory Peck in *The*

total trend-setter

During the twenties and early thirties, nobody set trends in men's fashion like the Prince of Wales, to the point that British and American menswear manufacturers turned to him as a pacesetter. For example, brown suede shoes were considered vulgar and red ties effeminate until the Prince wore them. He single-handedly relieved a Depression affecting the Shetland Islands when he appeared on the golf course in a Fair Isle sweater. When the Prince showed up at Belmont Park, Long Island, during one of his visits to the United States, he was sporting a large Panama hat, which Americans hadn't seen in over ten years. The very next day, the Panama made a resounding comeback. He was also responsible for the success and popularity—both on British and American soils—of the glenurquhart plaid (or glen plaid) suit, a single-breasted number that he wore with cocoa buckskin shoes and a felt hat. The "English look" soon dominated both sides of the Atlantic, and suits with broader shoulders, wider lapels, loose lines, a moderately defined waist, pleats at the waistband, and snug hips topped the fashion charts.

Mix 'n Match: Play one style off another by jazzing up a pair of simple black pants with a colorful jacket, like this fabulous Lilly Pulitzer number from the sixties (left); or keep the mood somber and elegant by pairing the same pant with a tuxedo jacket with velvet collar from the same era.

stark raving mod *"Mod" fashions were born in 1957 with the opening of John Stephen's shop at 5 Carnaby Street in fashionable London. Virtually single-handedly, he took over the streets with his exciting new line of frilly shirts, colorful ties, and daring cuts, favorites among the young motor scooter group called the Mods. The look, epitomized by British model Lesley Hornby—better known as Twiggy, the beanpole figure with enormous, made-up eyes—was radically different from previous fashion movements. It was modern, unashamedly sexy, daring, and distinctly young.*

Man in the Flannel Gray Suit.) The days of bulky accessories were over, making way for slimmer ties and understated shoes. And towards the end of the decade, the shapely "Continental look," with a rounded, and cutaway front, peaked lapels, or the new shawl collar that makes for a softer lapel line, was starting to emerge as the suit of choice, making its true mark in the decade to come.

But thank goodness, not every man wants to be Cary Grant or look like him, nor does he have the ability to pull it off. And thank goodness for the sixties. Even if just for the options. With flamboyance brewing on Carnaby Street in London, and a new band called the Beatles about to set the fashion stage for the entire world, the tight-fitted "Continental" suit with higher armholes and a nipped-in waist made its début. Worn by the "Rat Pack" early in the decade, the side-vented jacket with tapered, cuffless trousers, as interpreted by the likes of Pierre Cardin and Yves St. Laurent, soon befitted every man and "modster" on the street.

With "wash-and-wear" appeal, the suit gradually developed a flared silhouette—both in leg and jacket—wider lapels, and a healthy cutaway front, revealing frillier shirts and massive collars. Owning up to the term "British look" or "London line," the suit remains an absolute, positive must in every man's closet. With less fullness and width across the chest, the smooth polyester blends are perfectly adapted to today's style.

crossing over

By the end of the sixties, men's designers were starting to cross over the fashion lines of demarcation from women's to men's. French designer Pierre Cardin was one of the first to open the doors and dive into the design possibilities in menswear. And in 1962, Bonwit Teller, the exclusive women's store, opened its first men's boutique, featuring none other than Pierre Cardin.

John Weitz, who originally designed for women and children, made the same leap in 1964, becoming the first American designer to create for men. Oleg Cassini (whose exclusive designs for Mrs. John F. Kennedy had earned him quite a following in women's fashion), and Bill Blass were soon to follow.

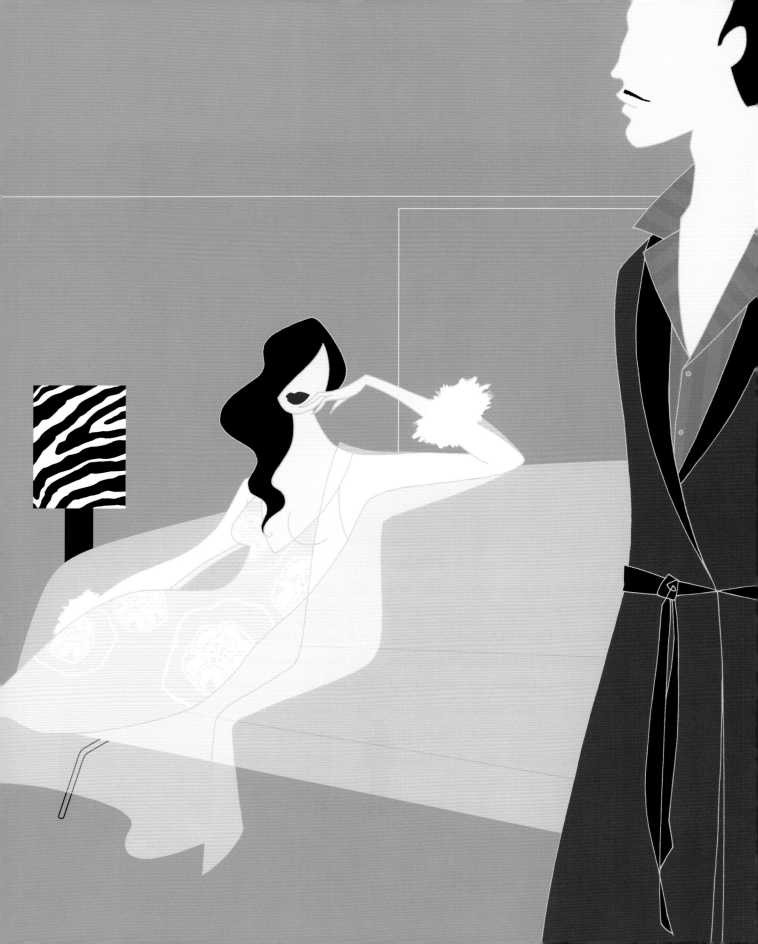

{5}

loungewear, sleepwear, & lingerie

"I base my fashion sense on
what doesn't itch."

—*Gilda Radner*

boudoir best-bets

With steamy Nicole Kidman catapulting corsets and garters back into the mainstream via the 2001 Hollywood film *Moulin Rouge*, loungewear and basically anything that has to do with the boudoir is sizzling hot. And it's also vintage clothing's best-kept secret. Because loungewear is one of the few clothing "groups" that basically has no boundaries (face it, no matter how badly you want to pull it off, you're probably not going to end up wearing a Pucci shirt at the beach or a peppermint ruffled-front seventies tuxedo shirt at a Sunday brunch!), there's no such thing as a bad time and place for it. Basically, anytime, anywhere works; for all to see or only you to know. Just ask Madonna. She single-handedly exposed the underneath of it all, back in the days when she strutted the stage in lace bras and golden corsets with torpedo-shaped

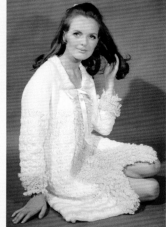

breasts. And it just hasn't been the same since.

Vintage loungewear, in particular, stands apart from contemporary garments because of its high quality and tremendous attention to detail. Today's newer fabrics just don't feel as good to the touch as the old ones do: remember smooth silks from previous eras, caressing chiffons, barely visible voiles, luscious satins, crisp cotton pajamas, and wholesome seersucker robes? And today's garments just don't exhibit the craftsmanship and detailing the old ones do: a 1920s lightweight French flannel robe with exceptionally broad horizontal stripes and a heavily fringed tie-sash; an embroidered fifties bed jacket with tricot trim and a ribbon-tie closure; or a delicate lace peignoir from the 1930s trimmed with an oversized pink satin bow in the back and tiny satin roses on the lapel.

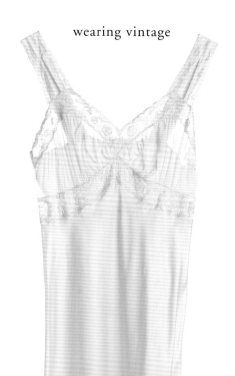
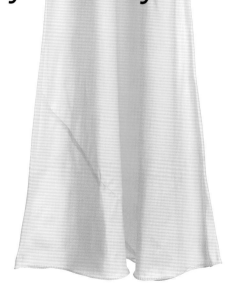

"Today's garments just don't exhibit the craftsmanship and detailing that yesterday's do."

A 1940s peach silk bias-cut nightgown with V-neckline and lace detail. Opposite: Some sixties bed jackets, like this knit one edged with pale green loops, are just too good for the bedroom.

{women's loungewear}

"Silky, sensational, seductive, and sinfully hot: vintage nightgowns, negligees, slips, night dresses, pajamas, lounging robes, peignoirs, petticoats, crinolines, bed jackets, camisoles, tap pants, teddies, and baby dolls. One for every occasion; two for every night of the week."

For centuries, women have been sporting undergarments that ran the gamut in terms of purpose, look, and appeal. From the rib-crushing "metal" cages into which Catherine de Médicis (the political and fashion diva of the sixteenth century) was particularly fond of squeezing her thirteen-inch waist to the slinky white satin peignoirs reminiscent of the one Jean Harlowe wore in *Dinner at Eight*, chances are you won't be able to tell what on earth it is you're pulling out when you dip your hand into the bin! Even after you try it on, you may not be quite sure what to make of it. But who cares? If you have no clue as to whether it's a slip, a sexy nightgown, or a little summer dress, wing it. What matters is how you layer it, frill it up, or tone it down; what spin you cast on it. Just think what a little fun, flair, and attitude can do to a housecoat.

eye-catchers!

When sifting through boxes of satins, laces, silks, and voiles, keep your eyes peeled for any of the following. And when you snag a lovely nightgown, always remember to look for the matching robe or bed jacket that might be hiding somewhere else in the store.

Fifties quilted rayon bed jackets with pearl buttons and lace trim; satin-striped nightgowns cut on the bias, in peach, pink, or light blue; slips trimmed with exquisite lace, fancy eyelets, embroidery, and appliqués. (Other favorite colors include navy, yellow, Nile green, black and white.)

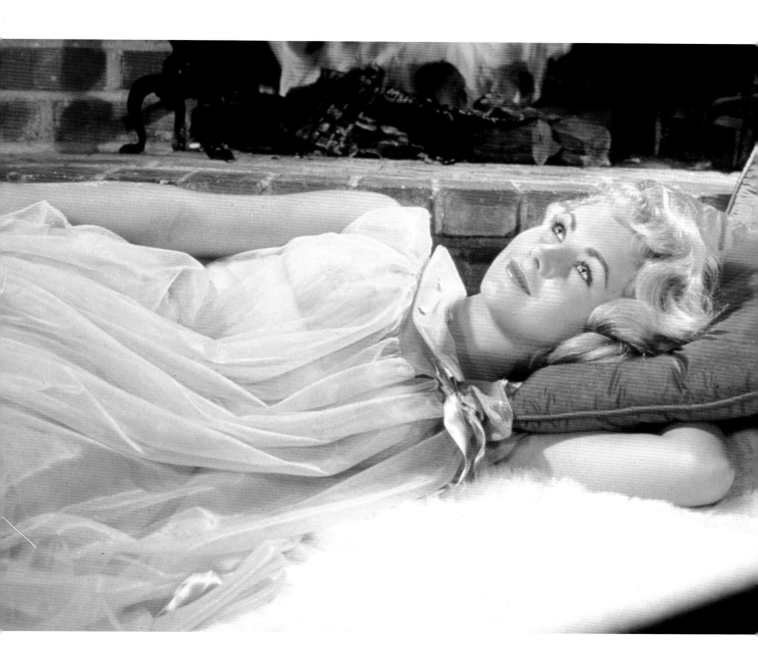

Indulge in a bit of yuletide daydreaming in a silk charmeuse nightdress with satin tie.

{nightgowns}

It wasn't until the 1500s that women stopped sleeping in the nude. For an extended period of time thereafter, they opted for a basic chemise, something akin to a shapeless potato sack but more comfortable. At the beginning of the twentieth century, however, sleepwear started to become more stylized and ornate as gowns and nightdresses made their way out of the bedroom and into the boudoir, the salon, the tearoom, the dining room, and beyond. Frilly tea and dressing gowns with details such as satin bows, intricate gold embroidery, and silver trimmed sleeves were for entertaining intimate guests at any time of the day or evening. In the 1920s, sleepwear had in fact become so popular that manufacturers were making bed linens and travel bags for toiletries to match pajamas and gowns.

In the 1930s and 1940s, nightgowns were formfitting and very revealing. They looked very much like eveningwear from the same period. Cut on the bias, with plunging necklines and sexy slits running up the sides, nightgowns were fashioned from such transparent materials as georgette, voile, and chiffon. When in the company of others, they were worn with fetching cover-ups: silk bed jackets or boleros, velvet capes, and luxurious wraps.

During the leaner war years, when fabric was rationed and women opted for more practical sleepwear styles like boy-cut pajama step-ins with buttons and front zippers, nightgowns briefly lost some of their frills in favor of function. Warmer materials, long sleeves, and hoods took precedence over coquettish sex appeal.

But at the end of World War II, the pendulum of femininity once again swung back, paving the way for ribbons, lace, lamé collars, ruffles, and sashes. By the mid 1950s, lingerie—and nightgowns in particular—had gone Hollywood. Actresses swanned around the silver screen in the most daring negligees featuring sheer, pleated

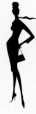 **more eye-catchers!** *Filmy and lacy sleepwear from the 1960s. Ruffle-trimmed peignoirs and leopard-print anything (and here's to you, Mrs. Robinson). Slinky white satin gowns and peignoirs with maribou feather trim and crystal buttons.*

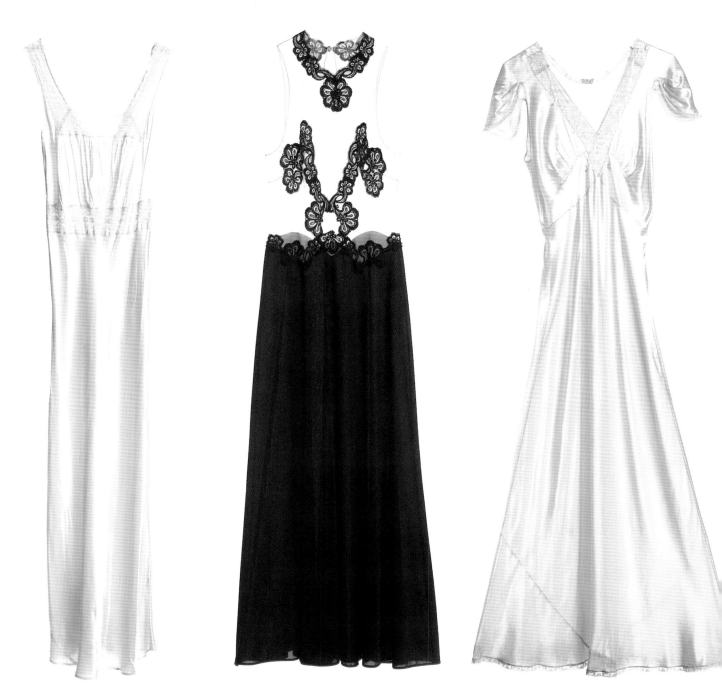

Slinky, sexy, and seductive with delicate lace detail and embroidery, these 1940s nightgowns could just as easily enjoy a night out on the town as an evening in.

ruffles and adorned their evening attire with chunky costume jewelry emphasizing visible cleavage. Sleepwear seemed to move with ease out of the boudoir and into polite company, blending in with evening fashion that carried the look out to dinner, to parties, and to the opera.

With radical times, sixties upheaval, and social emancipation came sweeping changes in bedtime fashion. Dramatic nightdresses from the previous decade gave way to short, frilly nylon pieces like the girlishly glamorous babydoll nightie. These revealed parts of the anatomy—like the upper thigh—that had never before been exposed. Thanks to improved manufacturing and fabric-dying techniques, wild prints in exotic colors like shocking pink, turquoise, peach, and lime green were all the rage. Short, quilted robes with extravagant borders and finishes paired nicely with shorter nightgown lengths.

The babydoll craze continued into the seventies, and they were worn *au naturel* or with matching briefs and lacy panties. Toward mid-decade, however, the enthusiasm died down in favor of an earthier look, what some began to call "unisex." Simple designs, free of intricate detail and frou-frou, natural fibers (cotton, wool, and silk) in subdued natural tones like cream, tan, white, black, and pale pink emphasized coziness and comfort over seductiveness.

During vintage forays, it's not uncommon to come across sleepwear items from decades past. While it can be tricky to find a 1920s or 1930s dress in impeccable shape, it's not unusual to find a nightdress from that period that shows minimum wear. Because sleepwear was exposed less to the outside world than streetwear, and because it was considered "special" and often kept pristine in a drawer rather than pressed into regular use, it's possible that the piece you find will have withstood the ravages of time just beautifully.

That's not to say that these ravishing nightgowns don't deserve to be taken out a bit more than once in awhile—and by out, I do mean *out*. Don't hesitate to layer a luxurious fifties negligee over a slip or underneath an angora cardigan and wear it to an elegant dinner gathering. Slide into a bias-cut nightdress from the forties, throw on a pair of mules and some rhinestone earrings, and watch the sunset at a friend's cocktail party. Or pick up a babydoll and wear it over short shorts at the next neighborhood barbecue. Whatever you do, don't just wear it to bed. Wrapped in the arms of luxury, you might never want to get up again.

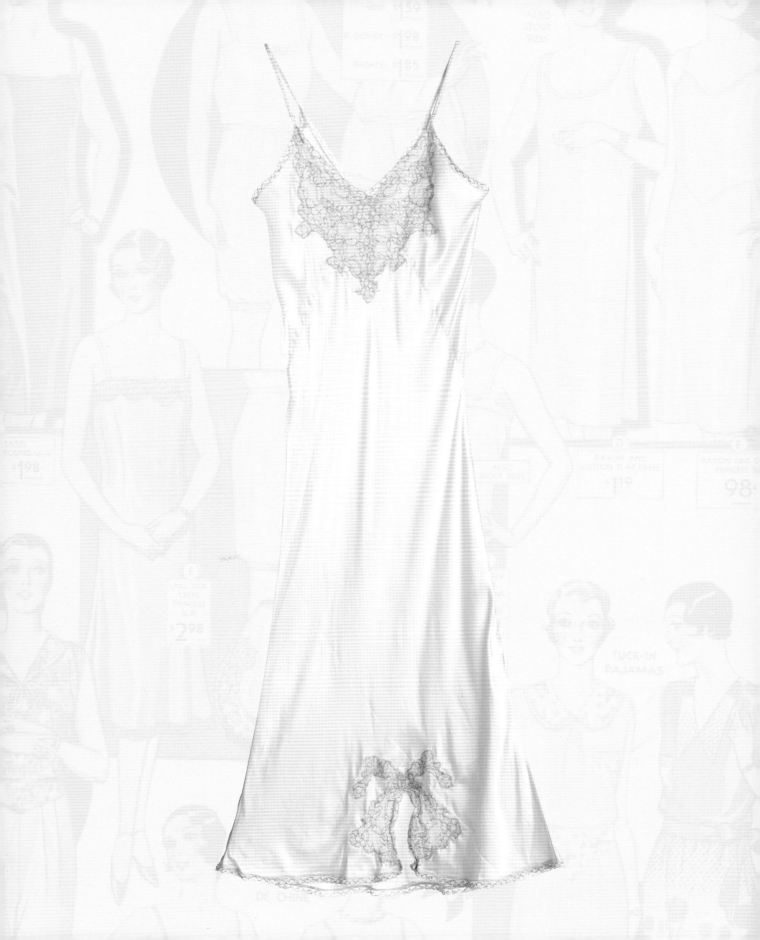

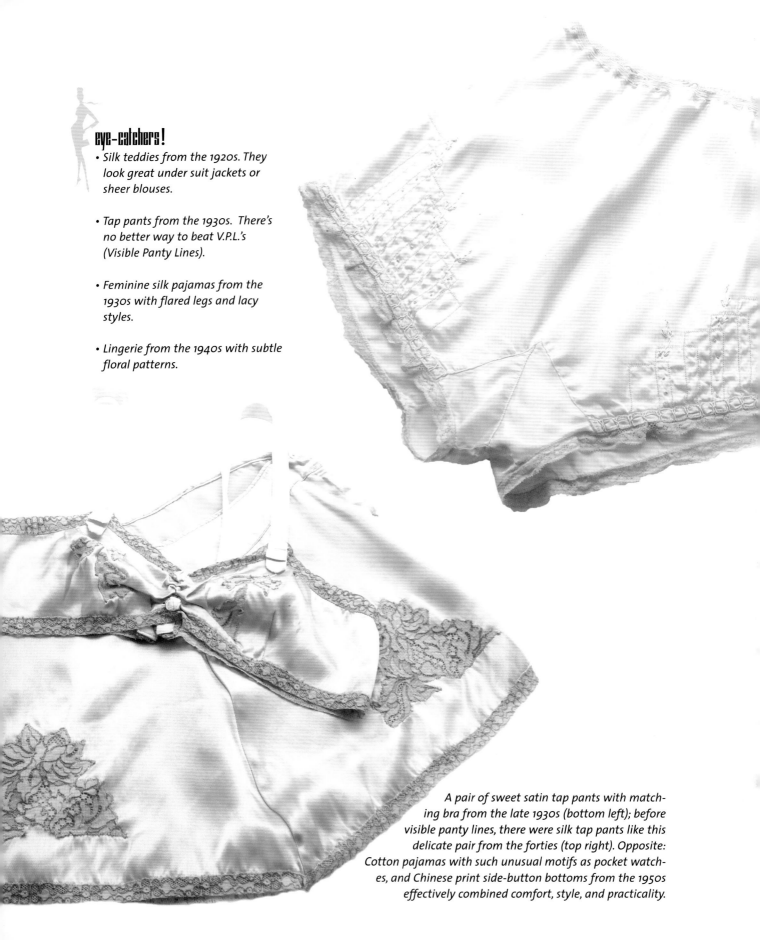

eye-catchers!

- Silk teddies from the 1920s. They look great under suit jackets or sheer blouses.

- Tap pants from the 1930s. There's no better way to beat V.P.L.'s (Visible Panty Lines).

- Feminine silk pajamas from the 1930s with flared legs and lacy styles.

- Lingerie from the 1940s with subtle floral patterns.

A pair of sweet satin tap pants with matching bra from the late 1930s (bottom left); before visible panty lines, there were silk tap pants like this delicate pair from the forties (top right). Opposite: Cotton pajamas with such unusual motifs as pocket watches, and Chinese print side-button bottoms from the 1950s effectively combined comfort, style, and practicality.

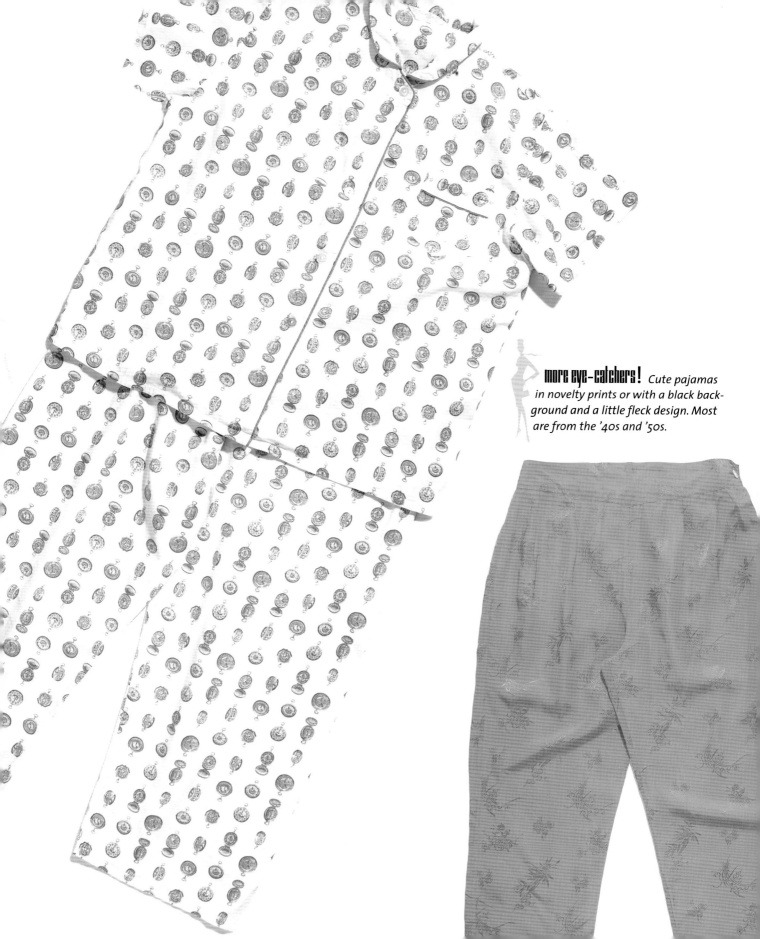

more eye-catchers! *Cute pajamas in novelty prints or with a black background and a little fleck design. Most are from the '40s and '50s.*

{bedjackets & robes}

Robes, bed jackets, peignoirs, and wraps became popular as soon as frilly nightgowns made their appearance in the twenties and thirties. After all, you needed something more substantial to cover up with in front of guests. And to keep you warm, of course. Just as nightgowns were elaborate in structure and design, with finishing touches that made them look more like eveningwear than anything else, so too was "sleep-outerwear."

A 1950s waffle bed jacket with three-quarter length sleeves and a delicate satin tie

Although these pieces were primarily designed with the boudoir in mind, it was not uncommon for quilted robes and velvet boleros to find their way into formal eveningwear and show up at social functions outside of the bedroom. Today, a belted dressing gown with a shawl collar and beaded cuffs from the thirties drapes as elegantly over a shapely evening gown as it would over a sexy bit of lingerie. A bed jacket with maribou feather trim commands just as much elegance at an intimate dinner party as it does propped up on a few fluffy pillows. There's also no better accompaniment to lean cigarette pants and a silk shirt than a 1940s quilted black velvet lounging robe with pink satin lining—and of course you can also press it into use when you need a little something to throw on as you run to the door to accept a flower delivery from one of your many admirers.

Vintage robes are just plain superb. No modern-day equivalent comes anywhere close to the warm coziness of a thick, floor-length, cotton chenille robe from the 1940s. A lightweight paisley housecoat from the fifties is ideal for those early summer mornings when there's a slight chill in the air. A short bed jacket with three-quarter length sleeves is simply indispensable when reading in bed, and a satin peignoir or a 1960s mid-thigh pink negligee with ruffled edges coupled with a pair of pink fur stiletto mules is the only thing you'll need when you want to feel like Doris Day in *Pillow Talk*.

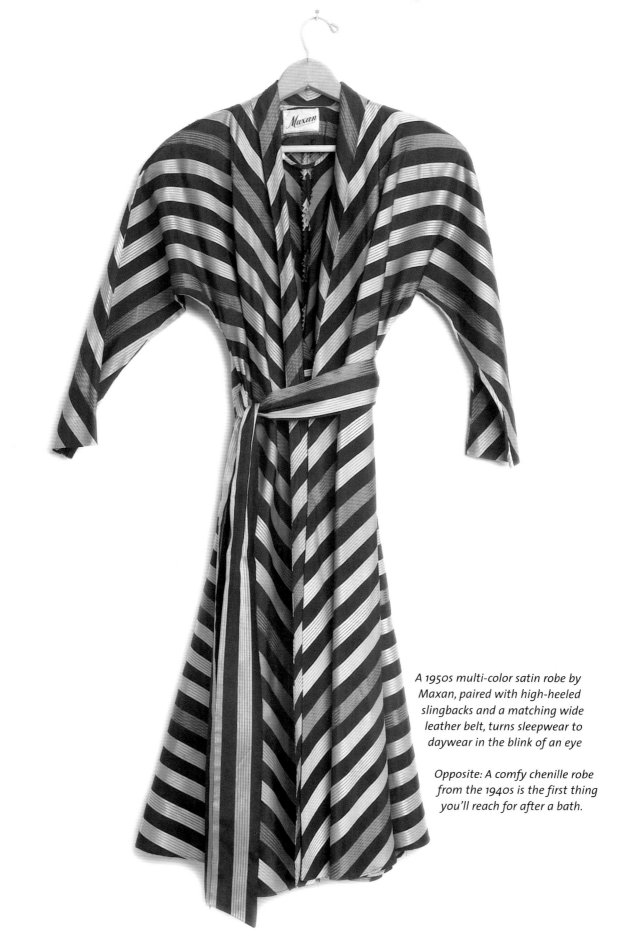

A 1950s multi-color satin robe by Maxan, paired with high-heeled slingbacks and a matching wide leather belt, turns sleepwear to daywear in the blink of an eye

Opposite: A comfy chenille robe from the 1940s is the first thing you'll reach for after a bath.

{pajamas}

Some vintage pajamas are truly works of art. In fact, it became clear very early on that men, clad in jacquard broadcloths, fine cotton fabrics, and silk blends, were going off to bed all dressed up. Pajamas from the 1930s through the 1950s, in particular, are the most stunning. Blazer stripes, awning stripes, and pajamas with buttons on the shoulder and at the side of the chest "Cossack style," gleamed with elegance and personality. Look for silk pajamas with patterns inspired by such sports as tennis, swimming, golf, and whippet races. Look for summer sleepwear in cool, almost translucent voile, almost as light as a handkerchief. Remember, "['tis] better to blush than blister. Better to be cool and vile in voile than vilely boil in flannel."[18] These summer pj's often feature extension waistbands with full-buttoned pants, and billowed pleats under the arm-holes for added comfort. Keep an eye out for crisp seersucker, whose crinkled texture creates tiny air pockets to keep you cool, and thin ginghams and sheer cloths with festive motifs: ocean waves, Caribbean shores, Grecian urns, flowers, and swirling paisley.

Vintage versions also include the coat-style pajama with convertible English collar, the pullover with notched collar, and the collarless middy, a sport style shirt. Some have colored or white pearl buttons, some feature knots and loops for a mandarin jacket look.

From the fifties through the seventies, loungewear was all about comfort and practicality. Full sleeves, full trouser legs, waist closures that could be easily viewed and examined, and wash 'n wearability. The sixties combined the best of sportswear and dress shirts into the pajama top. Henley necklines, classic crewnecks with three- or four-button plackets in the

the cats pajamas *Other terms for pj's in the sixties and seventies were the "unjama" (to emphasize its loungewear suitability), and the "kimojama" (a kimono/pajama combo ideally suited for the "new wave" man who thoroughly enjoys the notion of going from daywear to "early retirement" in the bat of an eyelash).*

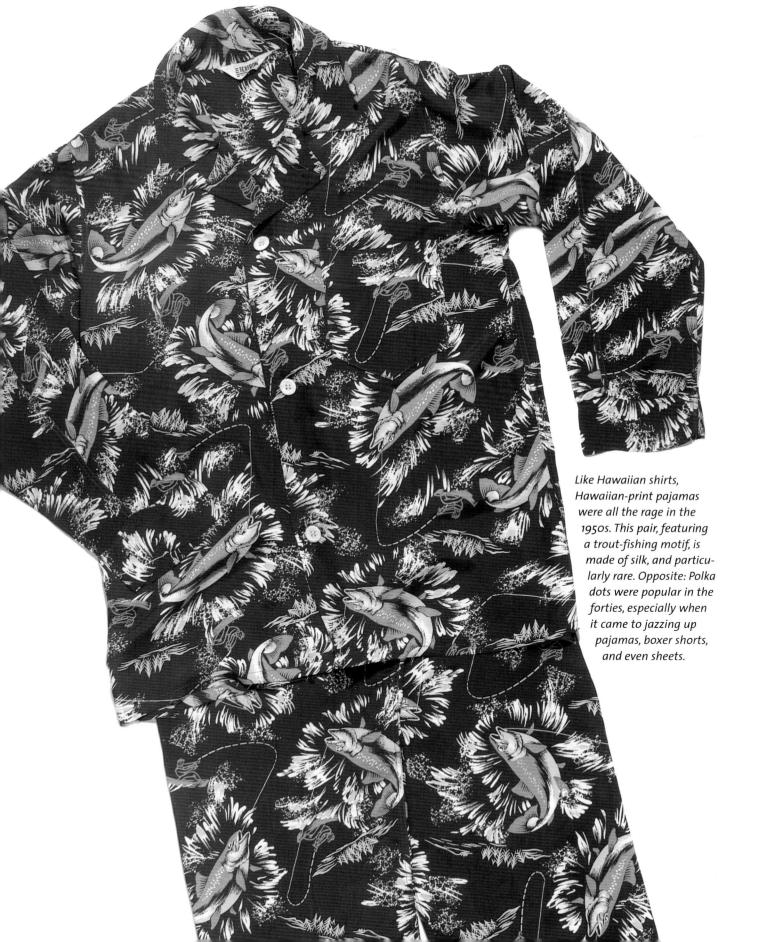

Like Hawaiian shirts, Hawaiian-print pajamas were all the rage in the 1950s. This pair, featuring a trout-fishing motif, is made of silk, and particularly rare. Opposite: Polka dots were popular in the forties, especially when it came to jazzing up pajamas, boxer shorts, and even sheets.

leg clothes

In the early 1900s, British colonials brought back a new type of sleepwear from India. It was called "pajama," which means "leg clothes" in Hindi. The loose-fitting bottoms had drawstring closures and were worn with tunic-like tops. The garment was propelled into the spotlight when heartthrob Rudolph Valentino appeared in lounging pajamas on the silver screen, capturing the heart of every woman on earth. Pretty soon, wives were getting them for their husbands, and the rest is history. Flapper girls in the 1920s readily borrowed them from their boyfriends, throwing "pajama parties" until the wee hours.

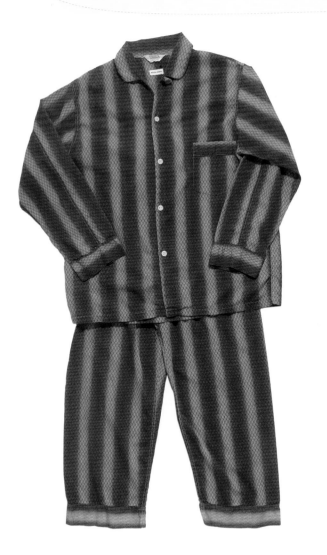

center; chambray pants worn with knit seersucker sleepcoats; button-front collarless versions of the traditional nightshirt updated to a belted knee length; simple cardigan pj's in bold British stripe. By the early '70s, sleepwear took on an even sportier, leisurewear character. Mix 'n match coordinate packages, sometimes in matching fabric and sometimes in contrasting fabrics and colors, swept the sheets. Sleep shorts of striped cotton seersucker with matching belted button-front togas, long-legged, solid color pj's in synthetic or blended knits with long-sleeved tops, three-quarter length sleeves and a sash. The nightshirt even made a comeback, this time in a knee-length model with long or half-sleeves, often in a printed or barber pole-striped motif.

Why settle for a T-shirt and boxers when you could be lounging around in comfortable Towncraft cotton JC Penny vintage pajamas? Opposite: Silk and stripes make everything nice, when it comes to this elegant pajama ensemble made in the 1950s by Van Heusen.

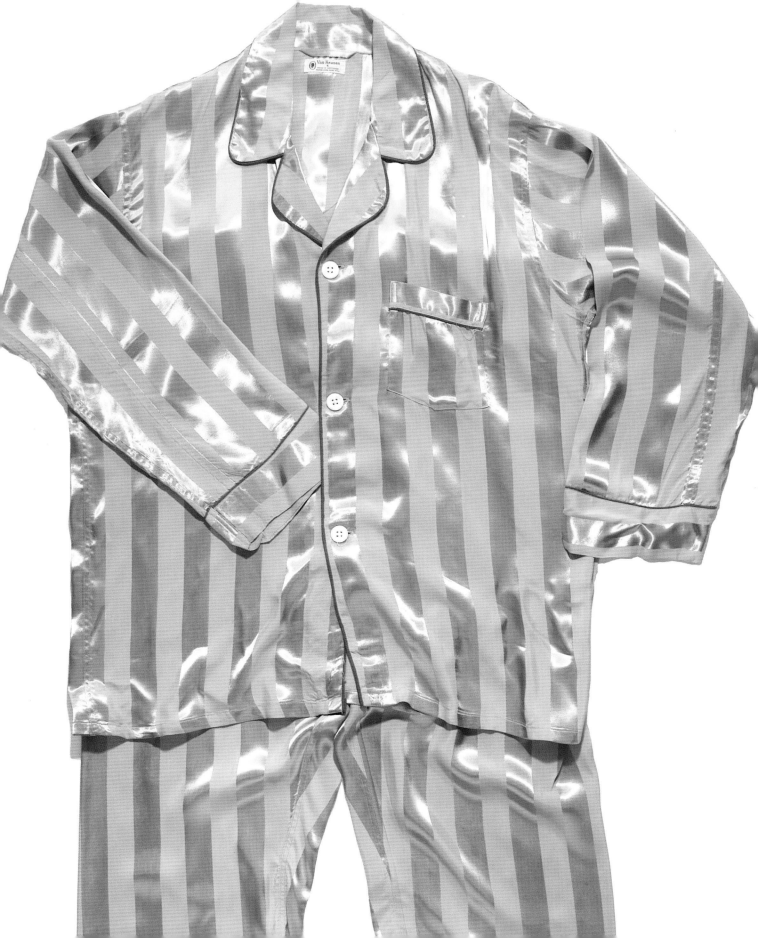

{robes}

If you somehow managed to get your hands on an ankle-length robe from the 1920s, then you've made quite the catch. These heavy silk brocade garments, usually with abstract or representational designs depicting everything from bullfights to Spanish flags in shades of gold, wine, purple, or blue, are some of the most luxurious ever made. Forget wearing them around the house. Take them out to dinner over a thin white or black turtleneck, show them off at the theater over a pair of slim velvet pants, or lounge about in them, provided you have a glass of the best Champagne in hand.

Beach robes—single or double-breasted, preferably with contrasting piping—gained popularity in the United States in the thirties and forties, when Palm Beach became the smart American resort. They were positively necessary when men dropped the swimming shirt, thereby exposing their chest hairs to the public for the first time. Today, there is no bet-

Surf's up with this Hawaiian-style beach robe with terry-cloth lining, made by McGregor in the fifties.

ter companion and cover-up for a poolside party.

As the importance of sleepwear merged with that of loungewear, the trend in the late thirties was toward fine tailoring. Woven woolens were imported from Scotland. Fine flannel, cashmere, and gabardine were no exception. Robes, cut and finished with the intricacies of cocktail jackets and topcoats, were commonly made in patterns of tweed, herringbone, or suited stripe. Patch pockets with flaps intensified the outdoors look, while slightly padded shoulders, yokes, and a topcoat finish heightened the streetwear effect.

The polo coat robe, double-breasted with wide, flaring, peaked lapels that added breadth to the chest and shoulders, a pleated belt-stitched back for fullness and comfort, was the "new look" for the forties. By 1950, a trimmer look in a variety of new man-made fibers emerged

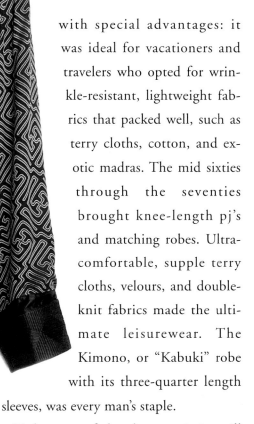

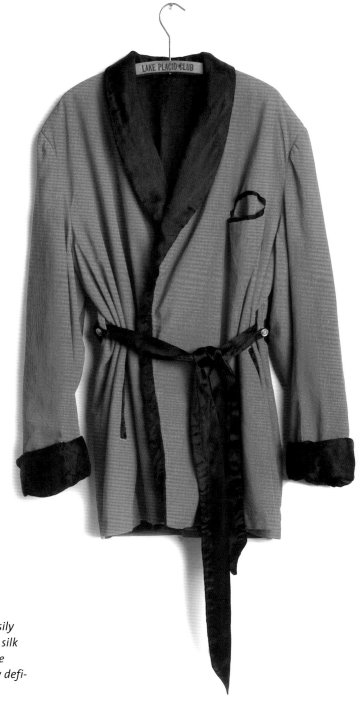

with special advantages: it was ideal for vacationers and travelers who opted for wrinkle-resistant, lightweight fabrics that packed well, such as terry cloths, cotton, and exotic madras. The mid sixties through the seventies brought knee-length pj's and matching robes. Ultra-comfortable, supple terry cloths, velours, and double-knit fabrics made the ultimate leisurewear. The Kimono, or "Kabuki" robe with its three-quarter length sleeves, was every man's staple.

Today, any of the above varieties will enhance the wardrobe considerably. Worn for their original purpose or paired with contemporary pieces for day- or evening-wear, you'll find out how easy it is to play Valentino on a restricted budget.

An elegant fifties smoking jacket with satin trim easily glides into at-home entertaining when paired with silk pants—or even jeans. Center: This beautiful vintage kimono-inspired silk robe by Ying Tai Co is the very definition of "mandarin" elegance.

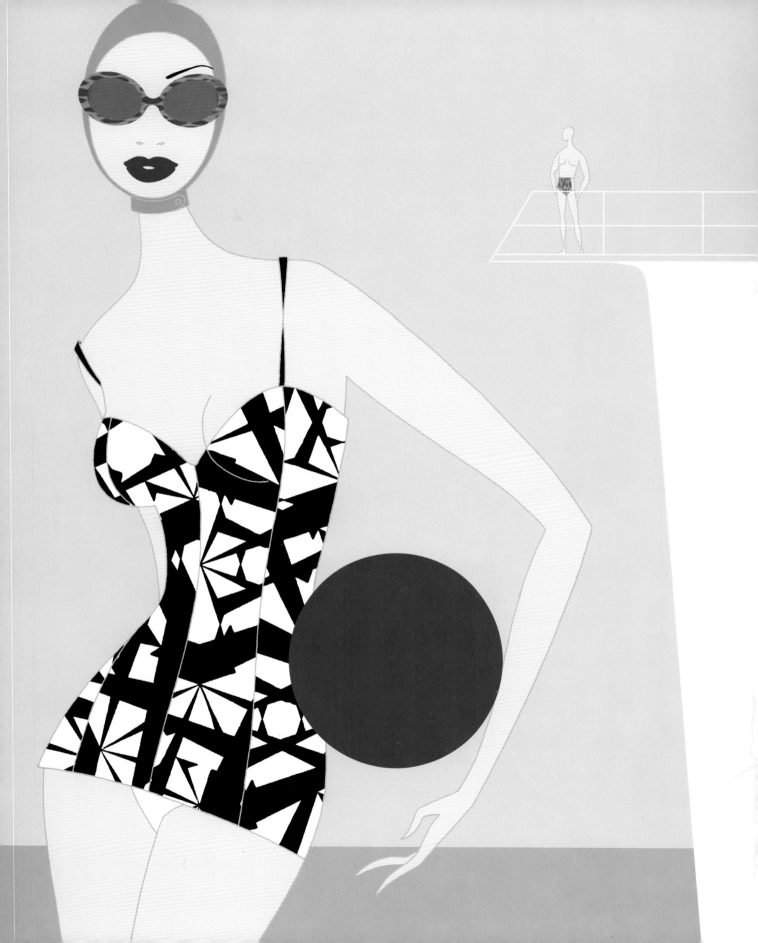

{6}

swimwear

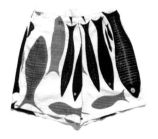

"Fashions, after all,
are only induced epidemics."

—*George Bernard Shaw*

making waves

If you can find a good piece of vintage swimwear, you've found the ultimate fashion catch. And there is certainly no better way to make waves. Few things are more coquettish than a forties swimsuit with a little flared skirt bottom, worn with a micro tank to go out dancing, or with its original padded top for a leisurely stroll down the boardwalk. A retro thirties swimdress, a fifties romper, an early sixties bathing suit in psychedelic or animal print, or a man's belted square-cut swimming trunk (à la Cary Grant in the 1954 film *To Catch a Thief*) with a groovy T-shirt, is the perfect companion for beach blanket bingo and barbecues.

And while you're rummaging through

Swim trunks never had it so good! Cary Grant twitches a thigh muscle in Hitchcock's 1954 film, To Catch a Thief. *Opposite: A late forties/early fifties classic one-piece with white piping by Jantzen. The company's Red Diving Girl logo caused quite a sensation when they introduced it in 1920.*

oceans of time and seas of styles, patterns, and prints, always keep a lookout for swimwear collateral (a.k.a. beach accessories). These include swimming turbans to keep you stylish (and your coif from fading) after swimming, daaaahling...(very popular in the fifties and sixties), men's beach robes or cover-up shirts, women's one-piece cover-ups or cute little shorts with matching tops, play suits, cotton muumuu dresses, halter tops, jumpers, rubber bathing caps with all sorts of decoration, raffia beach bags, mules with chunky heels, men's flat leather sandals, co-ed espadrilles, wide-brimmed hats, and—of course—sunglasses. And always remember to carry enough change for a Cherry Coke.

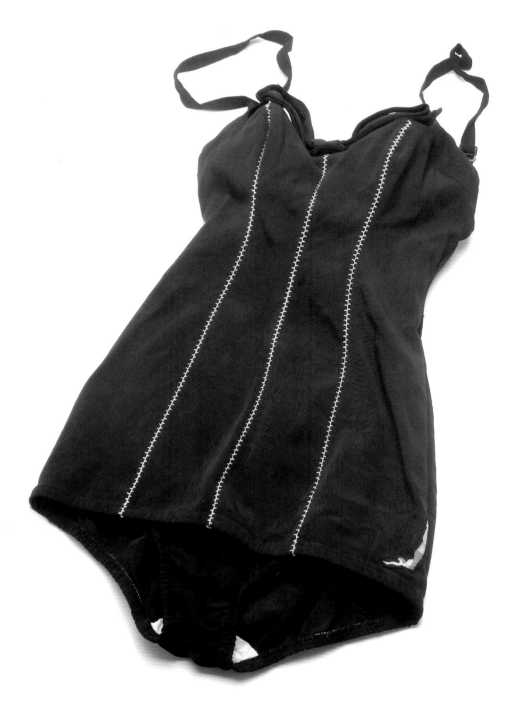

"If you can find a good piece of vintage swimwear, you've found the ultimate fashion catch."

{women's swimwear}

"Although you certainly can't dispute the advantages of today's quick-dry suits, there's something to be said for bathing—or just playing—in vintage glamour. Rhinestone buttons, Bakelite buckles, Lucite rings, sequins, ribbons, boning and hidden zippers for extra support and cleavage, will make even the lamest of fish come up for air."

Many women prefer the vintage cuts, especially suits from the 1940s through the early 1960s, because they're more "modest," less revealing, usually padded, and heavily constructed compared to today's skimpier standards. Those who feel they need more coverage and kindness for their contours and curves are delighted to slip into something Bettie Page, Rita Hayworth, Betty Grable, or Mamie Van Doren would have sunned in. Lower-cut legs, a nice hourglass shape that allows the wearer to be as big below the waist as she is above (if not bigger), and the added bonus of a skirted bottom are just a few of the many assets of classic vintage swimwear.

what to look for in vintage swimwear

Styles: Low-cut or boy-style legs, skirted bottoms, hour-glass shapes, drawstrings on the sides of the bottoms, constructed tops

Color: It's an important trademark of vintage swimwear. Black and white, or some combination of the two, are the most common colors. In the '40s, some styles were marked by dusty or muted shades of blue, red, and purple. Yellow and pastels became increasingly popular in the '50s; and of course, leopard print was so big in the '50s and '60s that it truly has become a classic. Black and white Greek key design trim along the neck and hem is a classic vintage detail.

Designers to look for: Cole, Jantzen, Catalina, Speedo, Claire McCardell, Halston, Rose Marie Reid, and Charles James.

Bathing beauty Esther Williams set the standard for aquatic elegance and grace in dozens of films.

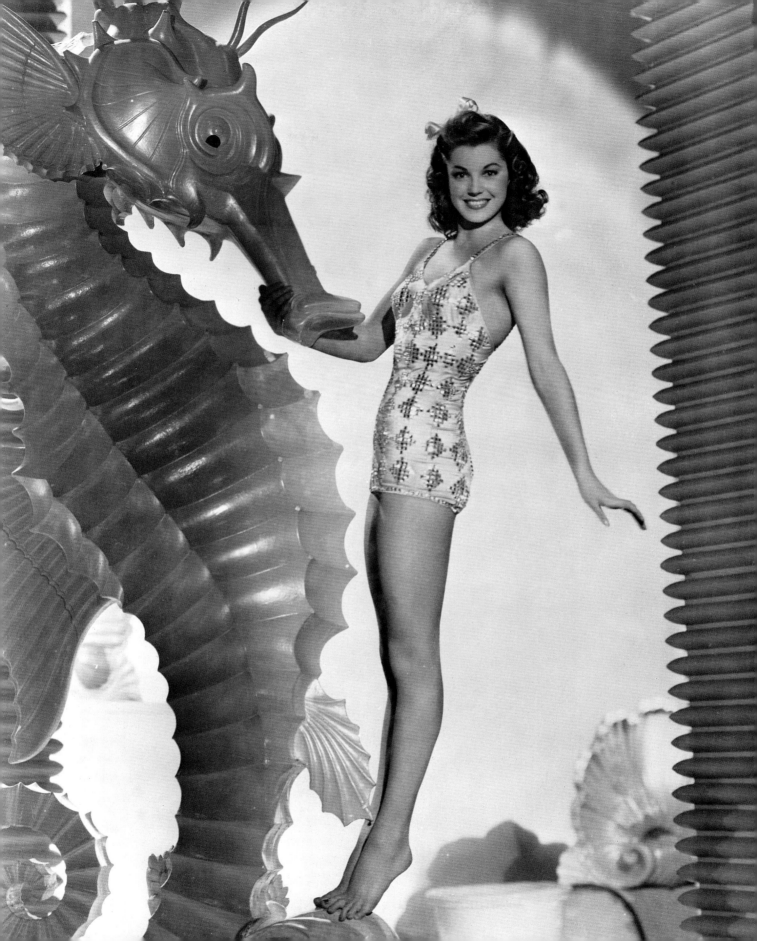

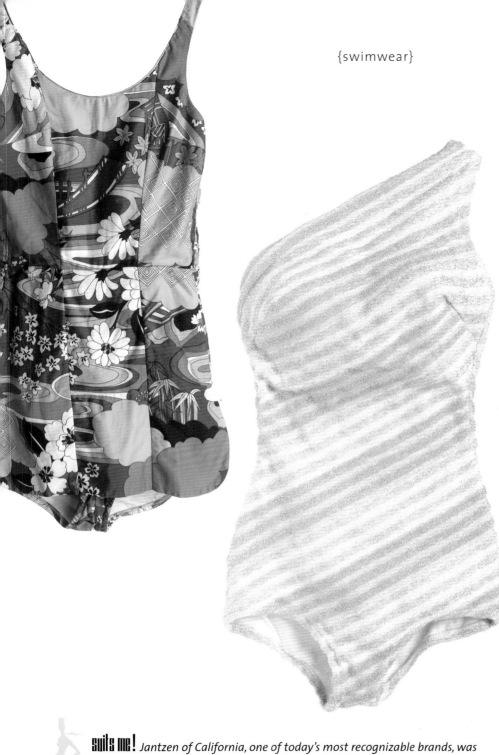

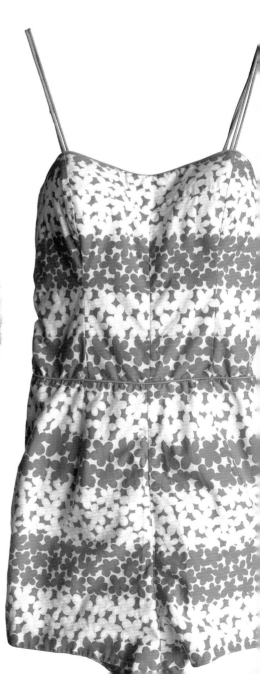

A parade of prints and styles from the fifties. Post-war détente saw a tremendous increase in the manufacture and sales of swimwear as more Americans hit the beaches. Opposite: This late 1920s wool suit with a plunging neckline, deep arm holes, and geometric details was quite risqué for its time.

suits me! *Jantzen of California, one of today's most recognizable brands, was one of the first swimsuit companies to rely heavily on national advertising for its success. In the 1920s, it launched an advertising campaign that featured huge billboards plastered all over Los Angeles and San Francisco. They featured a female diver in a red Jantzen suit, dubbed the Red Diving Girl. Pretty soon, people became obsessed with the Red Diving Girl, and cutouts of her pasted on car windshields became a hot collector's item. Jantzen then started offering decals of the logo until the Red Girl frenzy reached an extreme in 1924, when Massachusetts banned the decals from car windows. Being "Banned in Boston" was quite the promotional coup.*

Before you start assembling your poolside togs, check out old Hollywood photos and swimsuit pin-up shots. Think of the beauty queens from the '40s through '60s—Rita Hayworth, Marilyn Monroe, Elizabeth Taylor, Jayne Mansfield, Betty Grable, or Esther Williams in *The Million Dollar Mermaid*, to name just a few—looking fabulous in their conical tops and hip-accentuating suits.

There is, however, one slight caveat when it comes to vintage swimwear: if you're looking for something to actually swim in and not just splash in the shallow end, stick to the newer stuff. The reason is simple. It's a fact that anything

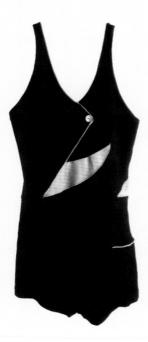

in the athletic wear department made prior to the invention of synthetics and stretchy, lightweight material is going to take forever to dry and probably weigh a ton when it gets wet. It actually wasn't until the mid to late 1930s, when fabrics other than wool were being introduced, that there were great changes in swimwear styles.

Synthetics, such as rayon, appeared in combination with cotton or silk. In 1939, Lastex, a rubberized yarn, was introduced and blended into fabrics to allow better "give." With the new fabric came a variety of new patterns and colors as well as new and different styles and shapes. Suits were cut

taking the plunge

In the 1930s, fashion was best known for its swimsuits, playwear, and beachwear. It was around that time that the trend began in California for designers to cross over from the world of fashion into the world of swimwear. Among the first to take the plunge was Hollywood costumer Margit Fellegi, who left the silver screen in 1936 to join forces with Fred Cole, the successful bathing suit designer and manufacturer. Previously, in 1925, Cole himself had abandoned Hollywood to work for his family's underwear factory. But instead of making longjohns, he started knitting sexy swimsuits. Flapper girls loved him because he dropped the back of his suits 19 inches so that women could get an even tan for their chic backless dresses.

lower in the back and in the armhole area to allow greater exposure to the sun, coinciding with the emergence of Saint Tropez and resorts on the Riviera as the new popular hot spots. Strapless swimsuits with an internal drawstring above the bustline were introduced, ensuring an even tan line on the shoulders.

In the 1950s, the impact of new man-made fabrics and fibers resulted in exciting developments in the leisurewear industry, particularly in swimwear. The new fabrics were light but warm, had minimum shrinkage, and were quick drying and waterproof. For the first time, elasticized, two-way fabrics were used in figure-controlling one-piece suits. Strapless and halter tops contained pre-formed or padded cups to guarantee the best shape. Bathing beauty Esther Williams wore suits so extravagant they could only be paired with bejeweled bathing caps.

A style that many women today look for and that contemporary designers are trying to replicate—a style which fortunately can still be found on the vintage route—is the two-piece, bare-midriffed suit from the forties and fifties. Originally known as the dress-up suit, the beachsuit, or the playsuit, its cut is youthful and fun, but still offers just the right amount of cover-up for a relaxing beach experience, with lower and wide-cut legs and a generous seat. The skirted look and boy-style legs, made popular in the '40s, is also an extremely flattering style. With a high waist and upper-thigh coverage, it's sexy and teasingly girlish at the same time.

Then, of course, if you've got killer legs and a body to match, there's the bikini. The itsy-bitsy two-piece number was launched by Parisian

padded for days

Suits from the 1950s are ideal for women looking for a bit more up top. Many of the suits from the fifties were equipped with convenient pockets to add the necessary padding, enabling the wearer to enhance her attributes if she felt she needed a little boost. Besides being made out of such elegant materials as silk, satin, lamé, and lace, '50s beachwear features many exotic motifs such as leopard print and Hawaiian backdrops. Parasols become the vital beach accessory and waterproof make-up—for total glamour, wet or dry—makes the ultimate splash.

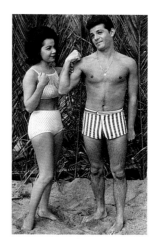

designer Louis Reard in 1946, after the atomic bomb test on Bikini Atoll. Although the bikini was a hit on the coasts of the French and Italian Rivieras—especially after British star Diana Dors appeared in her mink version at the Cannes Film Festival—it took another ten years before seducing American shores.

When private pools began to multiply in the suburbs, women started wearing the two-piece suit in the privacy of their backyards.

Of course, some women were resistant to take the plunge. Esther Williams was quoted as failing to see their purpose if they so easily came off in the water. That's when the convertible bottom was introduced. The suit was made to cover the navel, but had two strings that allowed you to adjust the amount of coverage. And then in 1974, the tiny stringed version made its way up from the beaches of Brazil and blew everybody out of the water. "Minimal" became key, and bikinis, worn like "body sandals," were straight-cut and tight-fitting with triangular cups. Halter straps and bottoms were designed to be undone easily from the sides. And at the end of the decade, extremely high-cut bikini bottoms revealed hip bones across the world.

One of the best things to do with vintage swimwear is to wear it anywhere but at the beach: at a picnic, a party, a friend's barbecue, for a quick trip to Home Depot, or anyplace else that calls for glamour and style. Fifties constructed halter tops look adorable with little shorts or capris, thirties or forties swim skirts worn with an oversized shirt knotted at the waist, a big floppy hat, some ankle-tie espadrilles, and large tortoise shell sunglasses (a must!), a seventies string bikini top with cut-off jeans and canvas sneakers, are truly the essence of summer fun.

Two beautiful bikinis from the sixties. Above left: a floral print suit with "convertible bottom" (side ties for adjustable coverage). Right: A groovy pleather original with plastic side and front rings.

{men's swimwear}

If you're like most men, chances are you've been sporting the same lovely swim trunks for the last decade. Maybe it's because you really do feel they enhance your best features and compliment your physique, or because you don't think anyone can tell there's a safety pin holding together the elastic. Besides, why spend in the $50 and $60 range for a brand new suit when a) you only wear it three times a year at most, b) you can get a new pair of jeans for the same price and wear those 365 days a year, and c) if it ain't broke why fix it? Well, gentlemen, it's no wonder there's so much sand-kicking on the beach these days. And there's a reason why Elvis didn't get any in his face in *Blue Hawaii* (1961), why Burt Lancaster managed to make-out on the beach in *From Here to Eternity* (1953), or why Frankie won Annette over so quickly. It's because they cared about their beach attire and

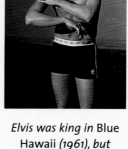

Elvis was king in Blue Hawaii *(1961), but twenty years earlier, Burt Lancaster sizzled in* From Here to Eternity *(opposite).*

understood that the limits of fashion do not stop at the shore.

That said, it's time to expand your swimwear horizons, and vintage is the perfect place to start, as it provides the widest selection possible. With what it would cost to buy a new suit, you can buy a handful of different styles from different eras, whether you're after the next wave as a Sixties Surfer Dude in wild Hawaiian print trunks, or the knife-wielding beauty Ursula Andress in *Dr. No* in a tight knit number.

A key moment in bathing suit history came in 1517 when the University Costume—a striped all-over number—was introduced on England's Cam River by varsity fathers who were hoping to spare locals' eyes from the sight of lewd bathers. But bathing au naturel remained the preferred wading outfit until the late Victorian and early Edwardian eras (end of

in hot water! *In Hollywood's 1953 blockbuster* From Here to Eternity, *the swimming trunk-clad Burt Lancaster somehow managed to battle rough surf and male arousal, all of this while successfully administering mouth-to-mouth to Deborah Kerr. Coming in close second was Cary Grant's narrow, belted knit number in the 1954 film* To Catch a Thief.

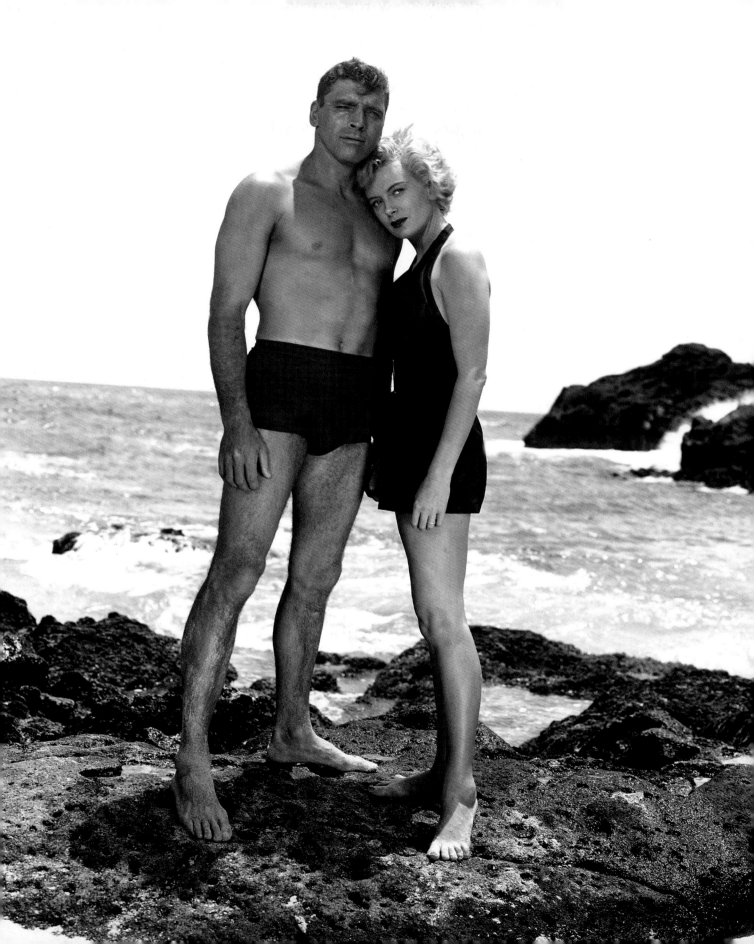

eighteenth/beginning of nineteenth centuries) when long, one-piece cotton or wool swimsuits were sported with Mr. Pringle moustaches.

As swimming evolved from a hygienic and medicinal necessity to a full-fledged sporting activity, men's swimsuits changed accordingly. One U.S. swimwear catalog from the 1920s described its latest poolside design as a "hip-length sleeveless blue and white knitted-wool top, low neckline and armholes bound in yellow, yellow cloth belt, white trim, white plastic buckle, fitted trunks, blue canvas beach shoes trimmed with white," and another offered a "one-piece suit with short skirt and deep armholes."[19] A skirt. Really.

By the early 1930s, the suit started shrinking. A popular menswear journal of the time commented that with just a few more nips, there wouldn't be a whole lot left of the swim shirt, let alone the suit. Halfway through the thirties, the one-piece number was shed for higher-cut and closer-fitting swimming trunks, coinciding with the emergence of the Côte d'Azur as the international playground for sunbathing hedonists.

Meanwhile, back in the United States, men were still getting busted (literally!) for walking

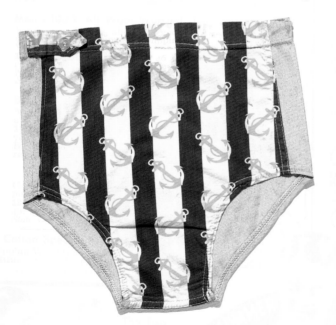 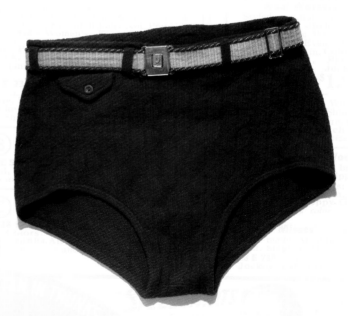

A 1950s anchor pattern swimsuit with an elastic back panel, and some very sexy Jantzen red knit wool swim trunks—complete with stretchy belt!

around with bare torsos and exposed chest hair, even up until 1937! But thankfully, things lightened up a bit after World War II, when pec-revealing trunks that started at the waist and extended to mid-thigh became the bathing costume of choice. Then, the square-cut knit boxer, a shape popularized by swimsuit designers Jantzen and Catalina in the 1940s (which, incidentally, looks great on heavier-set men), made its first appearances on California shores. It was an instant hit. But back then, unfortunately, the swimsuit had one major drawback. The boxer style, made from solid-colored wool, was often belted to keep it from falling off in the water. When wet, it was so heavy it turned its wearers into human anchors. Toward the middle of the decade, colorful Lastex and Hawaiian swim trunks were introduced and the swim top finally fell out of the picture.

With the arrival of so-called miracle fibers that were fast-drying and wrinkle-resistant, the fifties gave birth to a skimpier version of the boxer—a more neatly-tailored trunk—with extended waistbands and zipper flies. Some had pleats that made the trunks look like shorts, others had side zippers, and many manufacturers provided "cabana

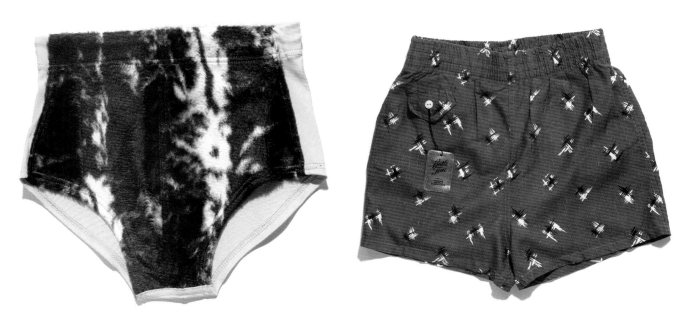

Grrrrr. . .A little faux fur goes a long way, especially on this pair of fifties trunks by Ganther. The more subdued Rustle Tone swim shorts with front pocket are from the same era.

181

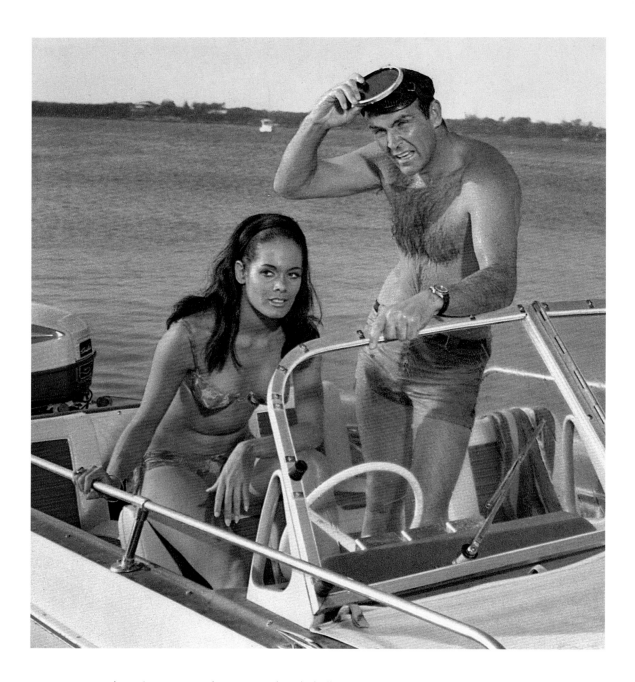

In the 1965 James Bond sensation, Thunderball, *Sean Connery did for belted swim trunks what 3-D did for the big screen.*

it's a miracle

The "miracle" fabrics that came out in the early fifties completely revolutionized the swimwear industry. With the introduction of Dacron, Vicara, and Dynel in 1950—three new all-synthetic man-made fibers—bathing suits could now be lightweight, crease resistant, spot resistant, easily washable, and durable.

shirts" to match the trunks. But by the end of the decade, there was a swimsuit length for every taste: from the low-rise bikini trunk to the Bermuda-length shorts and the short-legged Lastex trunks with a partial self-belt worn with a terry cloth cardigan.

The sixties saw Sean Connery as 007 in a belted, tight-waisted swimsuit that described the shape of his body without revealing too much of its mood. Also, as Acapulco became the new hot spot for fashionable resort-goers, snug-fitting suits in handwoven Mexican cottons were an absolute must-have. Denim, conveying a strong Western look, hit the beaches as well as surfer trunks, particularly brightly colored ones called "jams." They got their name from the loose-fitting legs and pajama-like concealed drawstring closure at the waist. Trunks designed after basketball shorts, with side vents and contrasting piping, were also huge hits. Pop art patterns, bold colors, wild

stripes and wide bands in terry cloth, corduroy, light cotton, stretch-nylon, acetate, and Lycra took over the beaches.

And then came the seventies, where basically the only rules were that there were no rules. With the advent of drip-dry, there was no holding back, and sometimes little left to the imagination. Some suits shrunk to micro size with Speedos (thank you, Mark Spitz) galore and bum-showing tangas from Brazil, revealing everything but religion. Nylon-tricot second-skin tanks—with few, if any, restrictions—provided total comfort, practicality, and fit. Belted tank suits with low-cut armholes (an updated version of the two-piece suit of the thirties) were all the rage. Even "hot pants," borrowed from the closets of American women, showed up in men's beachwear. Complete with studs, industrial zippers, and plenty of pockets, they look positively fabulous today with a cotton t-shirt or polo.

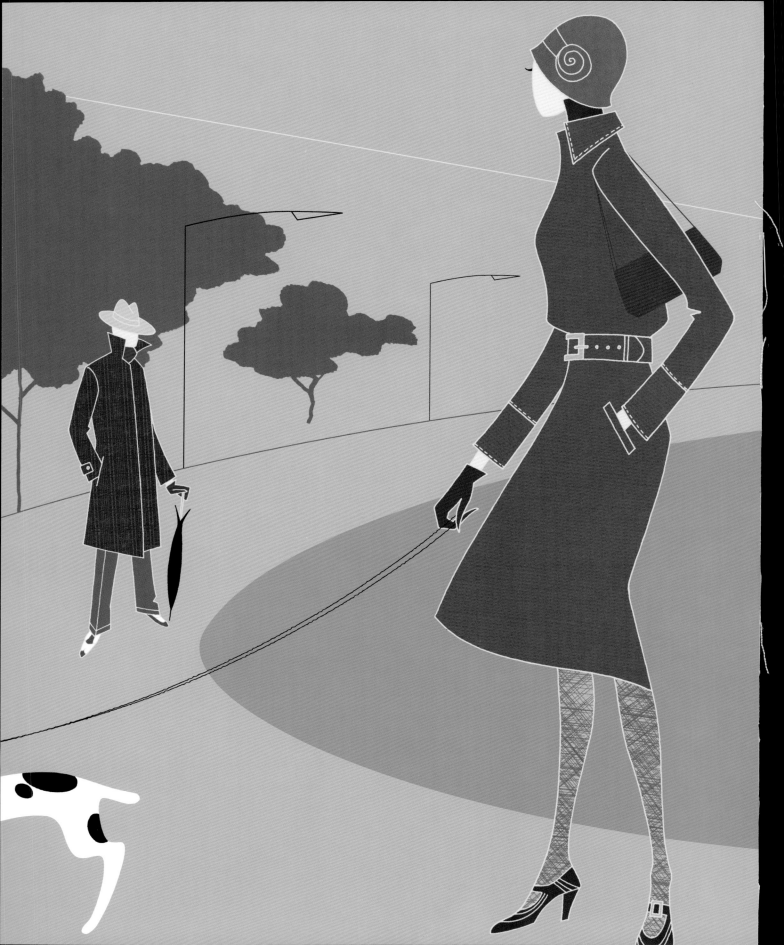

{7}

outerwear

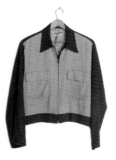

"If you are all wrapped up in yourself,
then you are overdressed."

—*Kate Halverson*

coat classics

Vintage outerwear is where you can get the best bang for your buck. Aside from the statement of the obvious—what styles! what prices!—vintage coats and jackets are made of sturdy material, since they were designed with Mother Nature's stormy wraths and winter storms in mind.

There are a few things to remember when you're looking for a vintage coat or jacket. First, if you're shopping in warm weather, chances are you're not wearing much more than a t-shirt or a light sweater, so remember to factor in additional layers for sweaters or a blazer when trying on outerwear. Next, consider all of the following elements individually: style, fit, quality, condition, practicality, versatility, comfort, and warmth. Once you've spotted a style that appeals to you and fits you well, conduct the "feel" test. With leather or suede, for example, you don't want

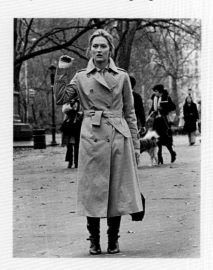

Meryl Streep played the quintessential Manhattan mom, cinched in a classic trench in Kramer vs. Kramer (1979).

something that's too stiff or cracking, telltale signs of poor quality, excessive aging, and improper care. If it's wool, stay away from anything that's too itchy; if it's fur, check for areas where the pelt might be thinning or falling apart.

Inspect the lining for tears and repairs; consider the cost of replacing it if need be. Tug gently at the seams to make sure there aren't any gaping holes or visible signs of distress. Look for detachable linings (a sign of good quality, especially in raincoats), removable collars, and interesting hardware like brass buttons, fabric-covered or Bakelite belt buckles, or small metal chains and fabric loops at the back of the neck for hanging.

And remember, if the coat or jacket is less than perfect but the style and price are more than right, you can always make some minor adjustments to give it new life.

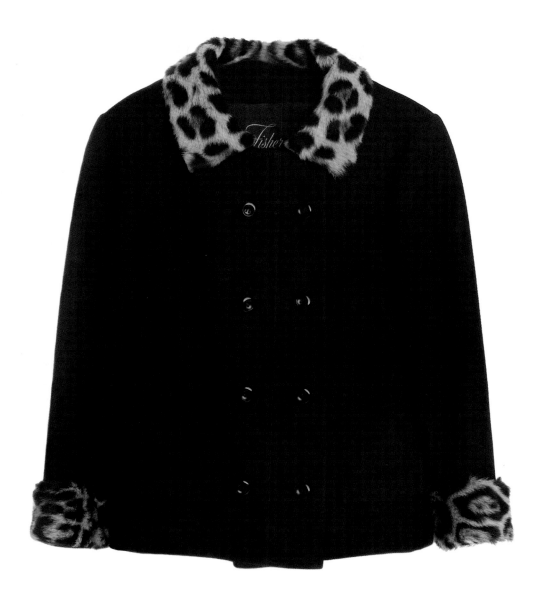

"The importance of selecting the right coat is totally underrated."

Leopard collar and cuffs add character and class to a short wool jacket by Fisher, circa 1950.

{women's outerwear}

"Select vintage outerwear pieces will do more than keep you warm: they'll have everyone wondering what fabulous fashion you have hidden underneath."

Some women have a fetish for shoes; others just can't seem to pass up a fabulous bag when they spot one; and others have a "thing" for coats. Long, short, maxi, midi, belted, double-breasted, fur-trimmed, silk-lined, military-style, princess cut, opera coats, faux furs, dusters, trench coats, swing coats, swagger coats, capes, and pea coats...when it comes to vintage, there's one for every occasion and for every style.

The importance of selecting the right coat is totally underrated. The fact is that wherever and whenever you make your grand entrance, the coat is the very first thing people see. It's the outer shell—the teaser to what lies underneath. How many times have you gotten decked out for the evening and had to "wing it" from the front door to the cab—opting for no covering at all and freezing your tail off—because the coats in your closet would simply not do justice to your gown? Have you ever taken your jacket off before getting to the coat check because you couldn't possibly let anyone see you in a herringbone coat over a plaid skirt, or a three-quarter-length coat over a floor-length gown? Or have you ever paid a small fortune for a trendy, contemporary must-have, only to pull it out of the closet a year later and wonder what on earth you were thinking when you bought it?

Well, that's precisely why you should consider vintage when buying outerwear. And it's really the only way you can justify having a closet full of coats, each with its own style and purpose, without experiencing any of the guilt. They're collector's items, after all!

For a fraction of retail, you can snatch an imitation Persian lamb coat with a shawl collar right off the vintage rack (or go for the gusto with a 1930s or 1940s

Meow!...A favorite of the vintage palette, a leopard print coat like this one from the fifties never goes out of style. Opposite: Fend off a chill (and possibly Big Foot) in a fabulous seventies fake.

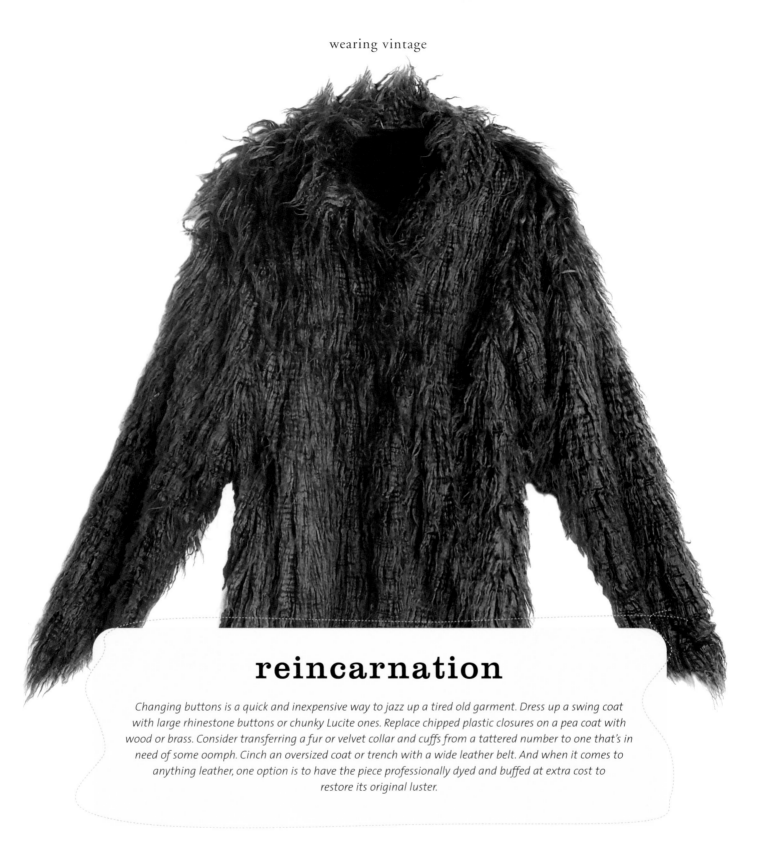

reincarnation

Changing buttons is a quick and inexpensive way to jazz up a tired old garment. Dress up a swing coat with large rhinestone buttons or chunky Lucite ones. Replace chipped plastic closures on a pea coat with wood or brass. Consider transferring a fur or velvet collar and cuffs from a tattered number to one that's in need of some oomph. Cinch an oversized coat or trench with a wide leather belt. And when it comes to anything leather, one option is to have the piece professionally dyed and buffed at extra cost to restore its original luster.

real Persian lamb swing coat with a large flip-up collar for a few bucks more!). Dig up an adorable 1940s poodle cloth wrap with a black satin lining, a 1950s sheer organza opera coat with a Peter Pan collar that fastens with a bow, a faux-fur double-breasted car coat from the 1960s, or a fringed suede western jack-

Skate away in an adorable sixties "skating jacket" with fur trim and felt appliqués. Opposite: Carole Lombard proved herself ahead of the feline curve in the early 1930s.

et (probably from the early seventies and worn in to perfection) and still have enough left over for the 1950s oversized man's trench coat, cinched tight with a wide leather belt, that goes perfectly over a pair of jeans and a crisp white shirt. (For more on trench coats, see Men's Outerwear, page 200). The bottom line is that while you might not come across Schiaparelli's original 1938 luscious black velvet cape emblazoned in gold sequins and beads with an embroidered rendering of the foun-

tain of Apollo at Versailles at your local thrift, or even Norell's over-the-top white evening coat of turkey feathers circa 1970, you'll most likely find something smashing that will complement your taste, style, and budget.

And remember to keep your eyes peeled for details such as the quality and condition of the lining and whether or not it's detachable; inspect the type of buttons used (rhinestones, faux tortoise, faux pearl, brass, Lucite, leather, cloth-covered, glass, wood)—sometimes the buttons are more valuable than the coat itself, so make sure all buttons are accounted for and consider the possibility of replacing them if need be; test all zippers and snaps; check for wear and tear under the arms and at the hem; and if there are belt loops on the garment, look for the belt.

Taking it! *The fifties was the decade of fur. Fur collars, fur cuffs, fur coats, fur stoles, fur jackets, fur hats, fur purses, fur shoes, fur boots, fur trim...fur everything. Leopard, chinchilla, mink, sable, monkey, zebra, shearling, giraffe, ocelot, beaver, Persian lamb, raccoon, alpaca, mouton, alligator, rabbit, fox—basically any animal that had a coat was in serious danger of losing it for the purpose of putting it on someone else's back. Things got so out of hand that Congress intervened (see "Fur-get It!" page 221) to protect certain species from extinction, and to implement strict guidelines and control measures for treating and handling animals and pelts. The sixties reacted to the excesses and the environmental disregard of the previous generation by embracing faux fur. From "mock croc" and leopard print on high gauge corduroy to "pleather," man-mades took over and pelts were tossed aside in favor of political correctness with glamour and appeal.*

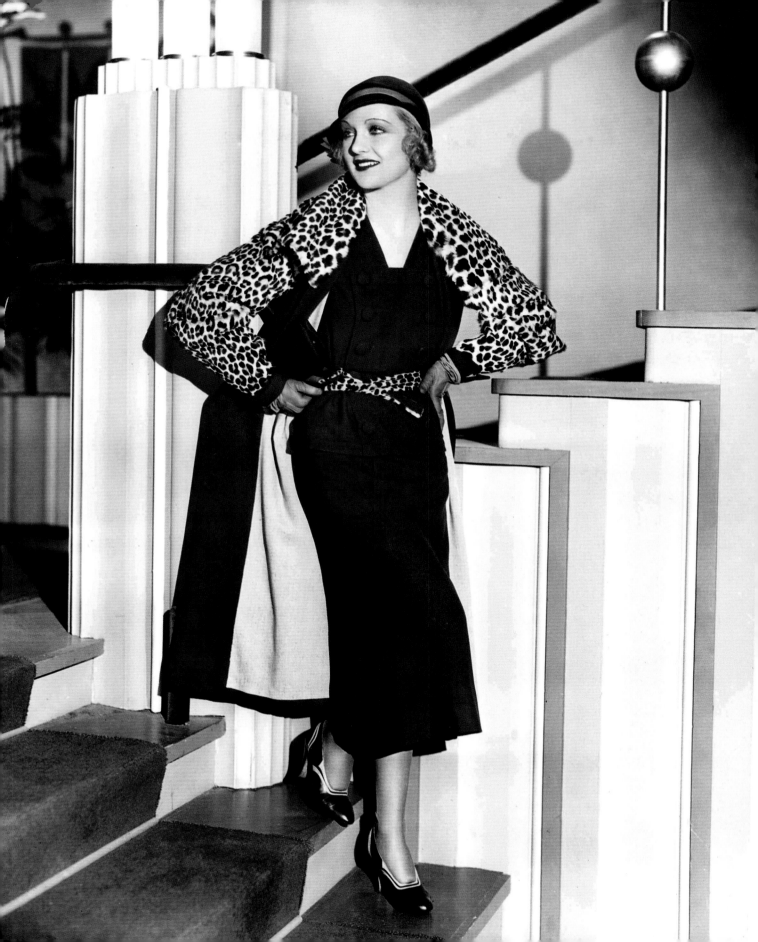

{peacoats}

The peacoat embodies classic outerwear style par excellence. It gained haute couture status in the 1930s, when Coco Chanel took the boxy-style, double-breasted, notched-lapel, blue melton, hip-length coat—an integral part of a sailor's uniform since the early eighteenth century—and transformed it into the veritable fashion gem that it is today. The peacoat gets its name from "pij," "py," or "pii," an Old Dutch word for a thick, coarse woolen cloth or felt whose origins go as far back as the 1400s. Peacoats were worn by the U.S. Navy from the 1830s to the end of World War II. Schott Bros., a New Jersey company that supplied the coats during the war (and also made leather bomber jackets), has continued to make peacoats, complete with anchor-pressed plastic buttons and padded lining. Pair one with slim trousers, a turtleneck, and flats, or throw it over a T-shirt, pleated skirt, and knee socks for schoolgirl charm. Sober it up with a cashmere crew neck tucked into pleated corduroys tightly belted, and jazz it up with a rhinestone pin or row upon row of Bakelite wrist bangles.

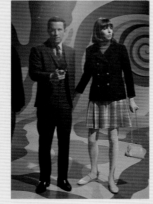

Agent 99 is super cool in her peacoat in the 1960s hit TV series, Get Smart.

nautical & nice

In 1924, Coco Chanel opens her first shop in Deauville, France, a posh seaside resort for the well-to-do and fashion conscious. She fills her little shop with knit sailor's shirts, striped sailor sweaters from Brittany, wide-legged dough-boy pants, and distinctive straw sailor's hats, all worn with a decidedly feminine twist. Coco herself popularizes the sailor theme (a.k.a. the "Garçonne" look), and cleverly couples it with a radiant suntan, courtesy of the French Riviera. A few years later, she adds the navy peacoat to her signature collection, as well as navy suits worn with starched white blouses and sailor hats. In 1962, Yves Saint Laurent hoists the peacoat to higher ground in the memorable collection that opens his couture house. Saint Laurent's version features gold buttons—rather than the traditional plastic ones—and for the runway, he teams it with white shantung pants and blue leather sandals. Almost simultaneously, French actress and timeless beauty Catherine Deneuve casually throws her peacoat over a striped shift dress and flat pumps, and voilà!, instant chic.

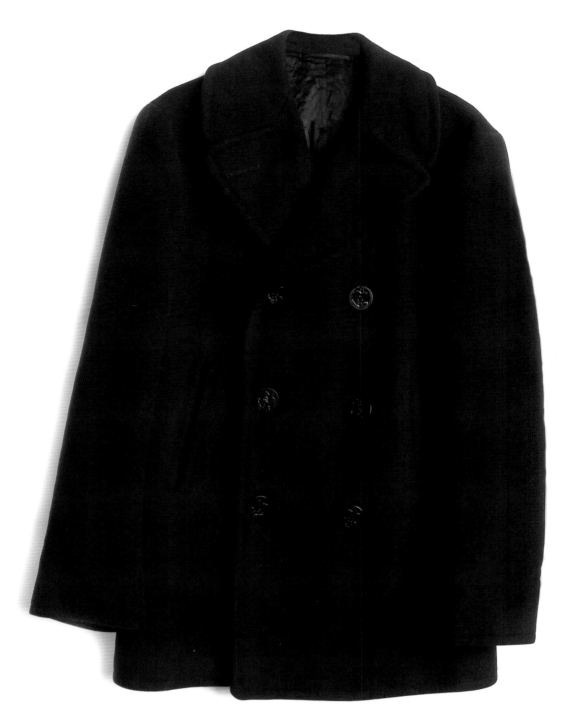

The classic peacoat: tradition, style, and comfort make it a perennial must-have.

{swing, princess, & swagger coats}

No outerwear wardrobe is complete without at least one of these gems. The swing coat is a 1960s classic. It was designed to drape over A-line dresses and mini skirts from the same era. It features a fairly fitted bodice and shoulders flaring gradually to the knee—and is as versatile as they come, complementing a pillbox hat or topping the bell-bottom trouser it was born to accentuate. This little number exudes freedom of movement; the coat's versatility has warmed and styled the likes of first ladies, London's "Chelsea" girls, and all-American hippies. The combination of girlish appeal with a show of legs makes the coat a perfect partner with short skirts and dresses, narrow pants, and leggings with high boots. And it's particularly flattering and flirtatious on women who may not have the height and stature to carry off bulkier trench coats and long, dramatic capes.

The princess coat, which was particularly popular from the 1940s through the 1960s and even into the early 1970s, is a coquettish garment that sits just at or below the knee. Slim, it has a fitted waist and belted back draped to swing below the waistline. The bodice and sleeves are narrow (with an occasional puff at the shoulders), and the proportions are enhanced by a dramatic collar or generous cuffs trimmed in fur, faux-fur, or velvet. The princess coat is extremely feminine and works best with clothes that are form-fitting and snug, so as not to interfere with its dainty style.

The swagger coat is a relic from the 1930s Big Band era. Inspired by men's military garb, the swagger is long, loose, and fairly unstructured, with the exception of shoulder pads and occasionally a belt. It's ideal for women who are tall or have large frames. Because it's a wide-cut and ample coat, it looks great with just about any style of clothing—short, long, tight, or loose—and works splendidly from morning into night.

A sixties version of the princess coat (above) defines femininity with its fitted bodice and narrow sleeves. The two faces of the swing coat: girlish, with a fifties' Peter Pan collar and covered buttons (opposite); and sixties sassy, in lined silk with gold accents (right).

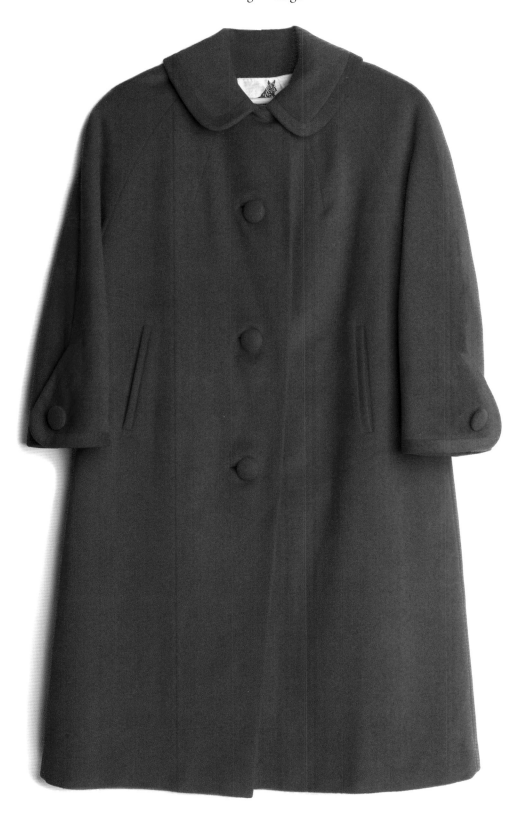

{the poncho}

Valerie Harper as "Rhoda," the hip window dresser, wore one in *The Mary Tyler Moore Show*; Clint Eastwood wouldn't get on or off his horse without one; and Ali McGraw's *Love Story* just wouldn't have unfolded in the same tearful way. We're talking ponchos, here: rectangular shaped blankets with holes in the middle for the head. They are seventies throwbacks made from wool, polyester, denim, patchwork, sometimes even suede. Almost all of them have fringe, though some substitute intricate glass beading and others feature grandma's pompom ball fringe around the edges. Well, poncho panache is back and more clever than ever. The perfect poncho sits comfortably on the shoulders, leaving the arms free for just about any activity. Depending on the material it's made from (satin, silk, gabardine, felt, fur, polyester) and the way it's finished, the poncho has many moods and can be worn over a variety of outfits. A cable-knit wool poncho with yarn fringe over a sweater, jeans, or corduroys, for example, is ideal for an evening stroll in cool autumn air or for apple picking in the country. A silk or satin poncho with glass-beaded fringe looks superb and elegant over a pair of slim satin or velvet evening pants, or a slinky gown. It's best, however, to avoid wearing ponchos with ample skirts or over roomy dresses, unless you plan on looking…a tad frumpy.

Hollywood legend Lauren Bacall envelops herself in style in this wool wrap—a contemporary variation on the poncho that blanketed the sixties and seventies.

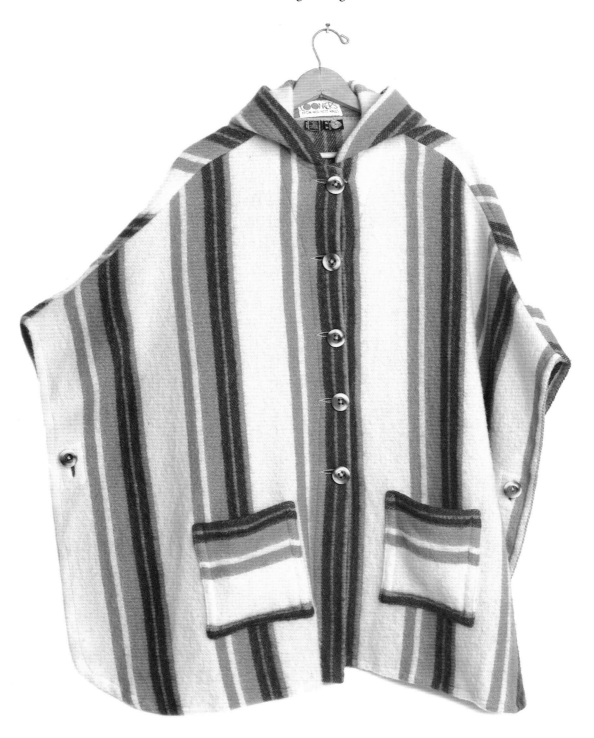

The poncho—button-down or crocheted and fringed—combines comfort and carefree originality.

{evening cover: opera coats, capes, & stoles}

Vintage evening outerwear completely upstages any contemporary pieces available on today's market. The reason is simple: whether it was to go to the opera or out to dinner, women just dressed up more back then than they do now, and vintage evening outerwear is a reflection of this lost elegance and extravagance. Coats were made to look more luxurious, often trimmed with rare furs and buttons made from semi-precious stones, rhinestones, or glass. Silk-lined opera coats and jewel-encrusted stoles made their dramatic entrances at parties and black-tie affairs on a regular basis, hinting at the fabulous gowns underneath.

Opera coats, roomy garments with a graceful drape and deep pockets, made their first appearance in the late nineteenth-century. From the 1920s through the 1940s, they enjoyed a sec- ond wave of popularity, followed by a third appearance in the 1950s. Today, more than fifty years later, opera coats are swiftly swept off coat racks in secondhand and vintage shops and ele- gantly draped over eveningwear for a night on the town. But they also work well over more casual attire. In fact, an elegant coat juxtaposed over a chunky turtleneck, a pair of casual pants or jeans, and boots can be a lot of fun and a refreshing alternative to a parka or a pre- dictable double-breasted wool coat.

Look for traditional opera coats with dramat- ic satin or silk linings in vivid reds, scarlets, and purples. Keep an eye out for brocade opera coats from the 1920s with ermine collars, and for those made of velvet and trimmed with fur.

Also be on alert for vintage evening capes, dramatic garments that make ideal outerwear escorts. Like opera coats, floor-length evening

Beg, borrow, or steal this luscious 1950s fur stole, perfect against a fall chill. Opposite: An elegant silk-lined opera coat in smoky navy satin, circa 1962, enhances a grand entrance to any black-tie affair.

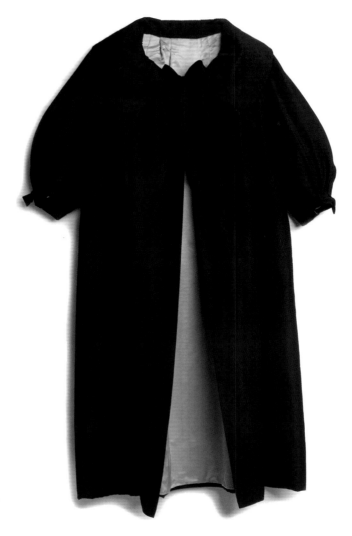

capes fit with the greatest of ease over just about any outfit, comfortably enveloping the wearer in a cloak of warmth, mystery, and elegance. Look for intact braiding alongside the edges, and for shoulder accents and embellishments like scintillating gold metal and rhinestones.

As far as fur stoles are concerned—fake, maribou-feathered, or otherwise—there really is no better way to glam up an evening. Swathed in a wrap of luxurious 1940s-1950s fluff, accentuated with a jewel-encrusted closure or a rhinestone clasp, you'll be positively unforgettable (remember Lombard or Hayworth's shoulder peaking out from underneath a fabulous stole?). But loosely draped over bare shoulders, don't expect too much warmth—except the glow that comes from all of the attention you're bound to receive.

{men's outerwear}

"Think beyond down or polar fleece, and explore the affordable world of vintage outer-wear, where traditional fabrics like donegal tweed, soft cashmere, rich alpaca, velvet, or mohair are the foundations for style and timeless elegance."

So you've got the classic camel or navy wool coat and the three-quarter-length weekend number—probably leather—and maybe a jean jacket or two hanging in your closet, and you think you're done. Wrong. You've only just skimmed the surface of outerwear possibilities! In fact, in the vast world of men's vintage outerwear, there's no excuse for an empty hanger. From herringbones to Harris tweeds, from beat-up leather biker jackets to quilted nylon parkas, from comfy "toggles" to double-breasted Chesterfields, the selection of styles and fabrics is endless. So why limit yourself to a predictable few when you could easily have one for every mood, or at least one for every style?

made for the shade

Among the many different types of fabric used for making outerwear, some of the more traditional ones include the following:

Bedford Cord: An extremely warm, durable, thick woolen material, often used to make sports outerwear like shooting and fishing gear.

Cashmere: Yarn made from the fine hair found under the coarse winter coat of the Cashmere goat.

Donegal Tweed: Coarsely flecked Irish Tweed.

Gabardine: A waterproof, wind resistant cotton weave with a characteristic diagonal structure, commonly used for manufacturing raincoats.

Harris Tweed: A popular kind of tweed, woven only in the Outer Hebrides, particularly well-suited for sport jackets.

Herringbone: An attractive textured wool in which the yarn is woven into a diagonal pattern, sometimes in two subtly complementary shades.

Houndstooth: A casual pattern that looks like its name, made from two tones of wool.

Tweed: A nubby woolen fabric made primarily in Scotland, woven from yarns of different colors. The name probably comes from "tweel," the Scottish word for "twill."

Vicuña: A very expensive fabric made from the inner hair of humpless South American camels related to llamas.

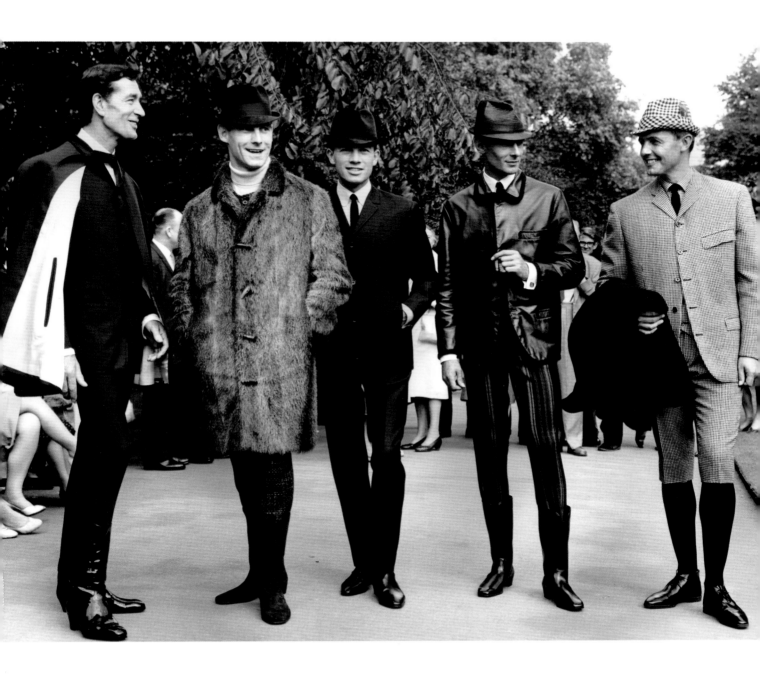

The sixties were responsible for some of the most innovative (and sometimes forgettable) designs in men's outer-wear, including the short cape and the mid-thigh fur toggle coat.

{jackets}

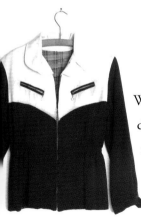

Whether it's a sporty lightweight gabardine jacket, a zip-front pointed-collar number from the early 1950s, or the coolest leather motorcycle jacket ever, vintage jackets are fun and versatile.

There's no better way to completely transform an outfit and douse it with extra character and flavor by throwing on a vintage jacket. It's the difference between going out with pants and a shirt (yawn), and going out in style.

the complete who's who & what's what of men's outerwear

You're not even close to being done shopping in the vintage outerwear department until you have at least one from each of the following categories. Happy trails!

Commuter outerwear: A knee length coat with a zip-out pile lining and a button-on pile collar, worn with a herringbone cheviot suit.

Dress outerwear: A natural-shoulder sports jacket worn with a wool turtleneck and felt cap.

Ski outerwear: A quilted nylon stretch parka, as much at home on campus with a change of sweater and slacks.

In-town outerwear: A British warmer in camel-color wool with a genuine fur collar, worn with a glen plaid flannel suit and a British-type raw-edge lightweight felt hat.

Stadium outerwear: A long corduroy coat with a pile lining that extends onto the collar, worn with a bold Shetland sport jacket, a button-down shirt, and Norwegian-type moccasins.

Action outerwear: An unlined golf jacket with motion and comfort detailing.

Beach outerwear: A summer parka in a vinyl-coated madras with a hood and push-up sleeves.

Indoor-outdoor outerwear: A suede-and-alpaca-knit coat (dressy enough for a cocktail party in the suburbs or a day in the country) worn with a sport shirt and ascot. [20]

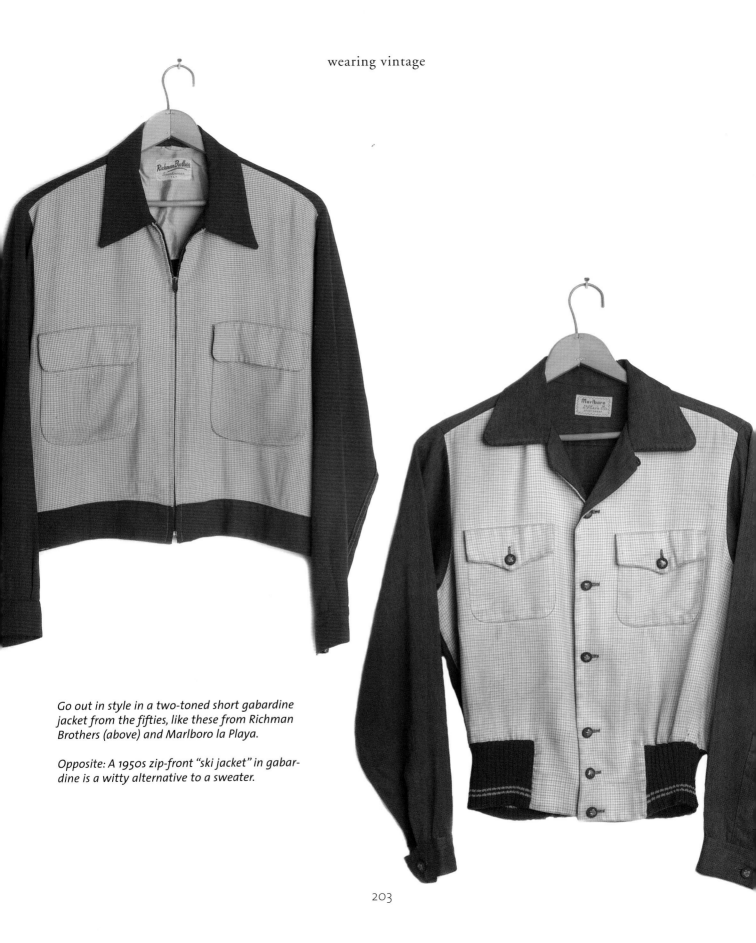

Go out in style in a two-toned short gabardine jacket from the fifties, like these from Richman Brothers (above) and Marlboro la Playa.

Opposite: A 1950s zip-front "ski jacket" in gabardine is a witty alternative to a sweater.

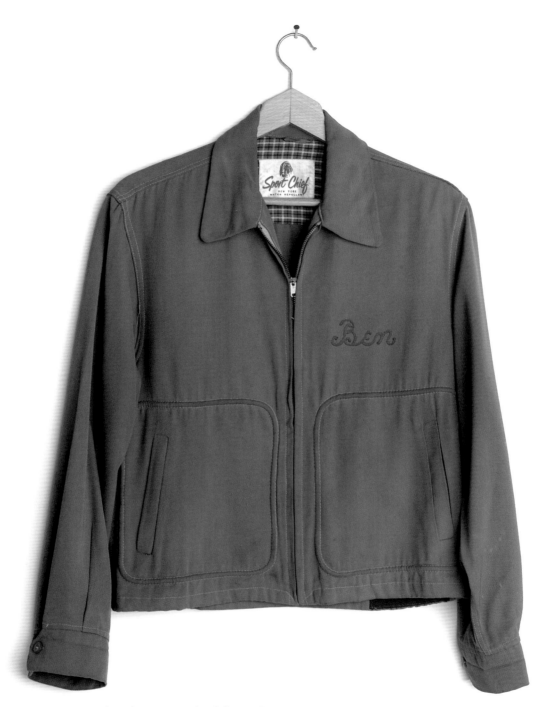

Another classic example of the zip-front jacket from the 1950s, this one by Sportchief.
Opposite: A stitched detail from the back.

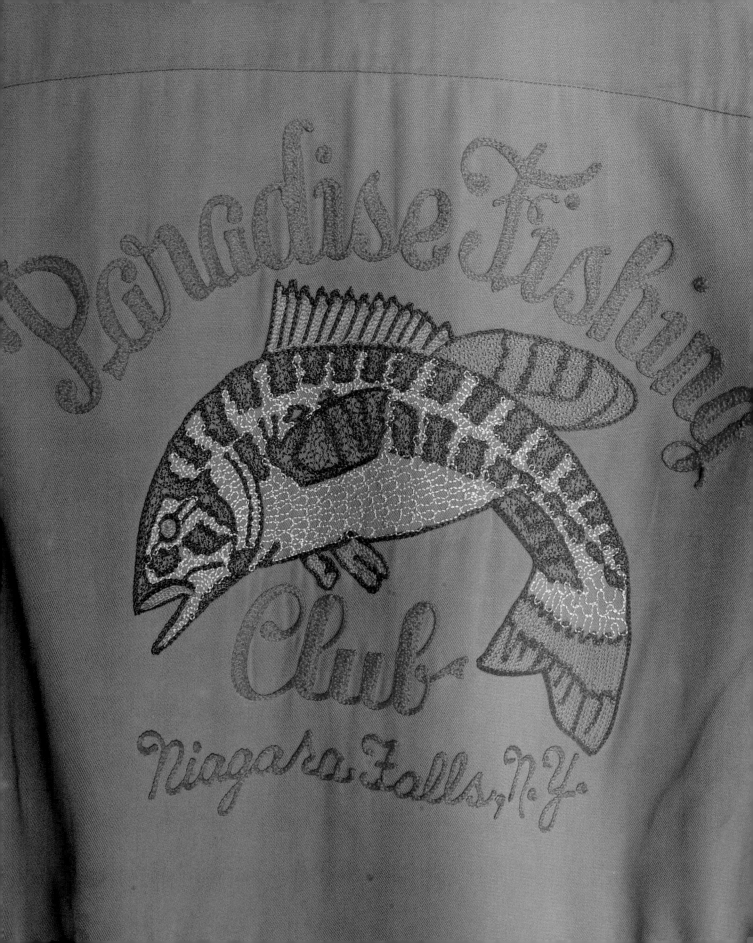

{the leather jacket}

Marlon Brando made it so sexy and dangerous in the 1954 film *The Wild One* that it was banned from high schools around the country. Chrissie Hynde created quite a sensation when she sported a bright red leather one on the cover of The Pretenders' debut album. And Fonzie snapped at anyone who came close to his in *Happy Days*. General MacArthur couldn't imagine leaving home without his, Cary Grant was the quintessential hunk when he slid one on, and in khaki riding pants, knee-high laced boots, and a brown leather jacket, Amelia Earhart soared the skies and made aviation history. The leather jacket has become so entrenched in American culture that it has earned a permanent place in museums, a space on the shelves of the Library of Congress (in fact, an entire book was dedicated to its origins and personality), and definitely a hanger or two in everyone's closet.

In the mid thirties, the sporty American man had a definite penchant for leather. The leather jacket came in all shapes, styles, and types: suede, horsehide, capeskin, lambskin, etc. Some were lined with sheepskin, others with raccoon fur. Some had large collars and deep cuffs, some were made from Australian wombat with a long-roll collar, and others were fashioned from natural china dog skins (closely resembling raccoon). Well, you get the idea. And naturally light chamois, champagnes, creams, light and dark browns were the colors of choice.

Buying a secondhand or "used" leather jacket is a no-brainer: leather is best when it's aged, worn-in, and smoothed out. It acquires character with years and attitude with history. And buying a leather jacket is generally a sound investment because leather tends to withstand the ravages of time even better than you do.

Leather jackets from flea markets, vintage clothing stores, resale or consignment shops

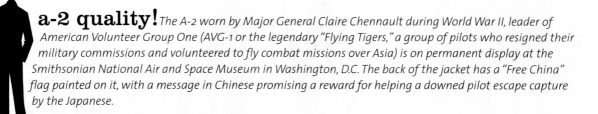

a-2 quality! *The A-2 worn by Major General Claire Chennault during World War II, leader of American Volunteer Group One (AVG-1 or the legendary "Flying Tigers," a group of pilots who resigned their military commissions and volunteered to fly combat missions over Asia) is on permanent display at the Smithsonian National Air and Space Museum in Washington, D.C. The back of the jacket has a "Free China" flag painted on it, with a message in Chinese promising a reward for helping a downed pilot escape capture by the Japanese.*

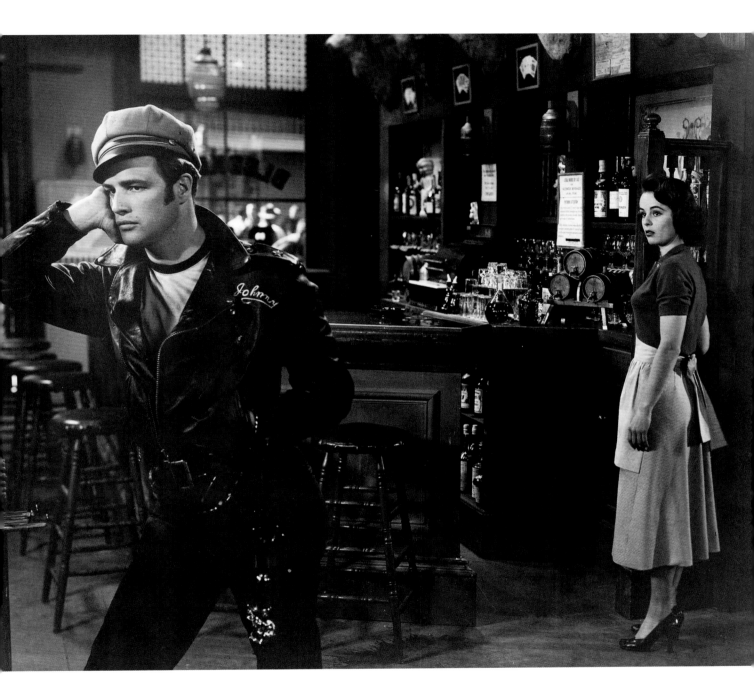

A brooding, leather-jacketed Marlon Brando is the very definition of cool in the 1953 classic film, The Wild One.

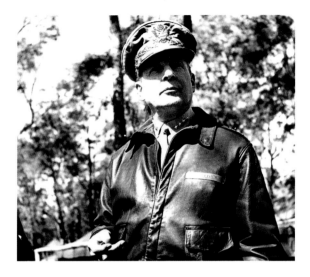

General Douglas MacArthur addressed the troops in signature leatherwear that was as ruggedly manly as it was practical.

the original mink collar and the original owner's airplane name inked onto the sleeve. Then you've hit the jackpot. When you're trying it on, remember that they're meant to fit snugly; their purpose, after all, was to keep a pilot warm in a cramped and open cockpit. Also, look for U.S. Air Force insignia where the zipper is sewn in at the inside bottom of the jacket.

Motorcycle jackets are another perennially popular style. The biker jacket is black and is prized for its thick cowhide, designed to help prevent "road rash" (biker lingo for the injuries from a nasty spill). You can distinguish a more

flying high

The first flying jacket, the A-1, was developed by the U.S. Army's air arm in the twenties. It was made from lambskin and fastened with buttons. The zipper was not invented until 1928. In 1930, Irving and Jack Schott, two brothers who began making leather clothing by hand in a small store on the Lower East Side of Manhattan, designed a leather jacket that they sold to the U.S. Air Force during World War II. Because it was so warm and durable, the jacket quickly became popular among fighter pilots on bombing missions, hence the name "bomber jacket." The A-2 jacket was standard issue for Army Air Corps flyboys until 1942, when General "Hap" Arnold supposedly pulled the jacket out of use, stating that the Army didn't need leather anymore and that there had to be a better alternative. Heavier B-3 bomber jackets were also manufactured. They were made from sheepskin and the outside was hand-coated with a brown paint mixed with lacquer which, with time, dried and cracked to reveal the lighter skin underneath. The most prized vintage leather jackets are hand-painted with images of magazine pin-ups of the period.

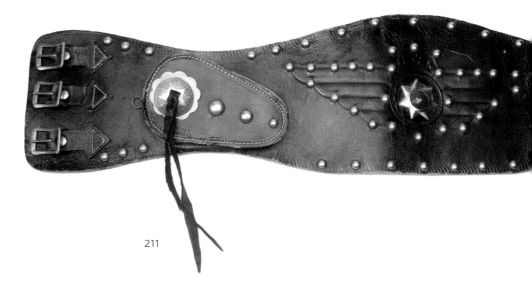

collectible motorcycle jacket from the forties and fifties from a sixties one because the older version tends to have fewer zippers. Some of the earliest jackets might even have wombat-fur lining. But even if the lining is beaten up, don't let it deter you from buying it. Although a jacket with its original lining certainly retains more value, a ripped lining can always be replaced with a cotton-blend material made for that purpose.

The Perfecto jacket or Harley jacket designed by the Schott Brothers, the original creators of the motorcycle jacket, was made popular by Marlon Brando, James Dean, and Steve McQueen, who sported them with rebellious style in so many movies. The first Perfecto, named after Irving Schott's favorite Cuban cigar, retailed for $5.50 in 1928 and was sold through Harley-Davidson Motorcycles. Almost thirty years later, James Dean's death catapulted the jacket into vogue and it retailed for $49. Today, a Perfecto from the fifties sells for $300 to $2,000, depending on the condition of the jacket.

The leather "Bronx" coat or car coat, the virtual uniform of the station wagon set of the late fifties and sixties, is another timeless, hardworking piece distinguished by its three-quarter length, boxy lines, comfortable and loose fit, three-button closure and sturdy, spread collar. The car coat—whose predecessor is the longer "duster" that drivers and passengers started wearing for protection at the turn of the century, when they were cruising around in open roadsters and needed protection from flying pebbles and dirt—is the perfect solution for warmth and versatility. Ranging in price anywhere from $100 to $450, the car coat looks great paired with jeans or leggings and a turtleneck or T-shirt.

Right: A studded leather belt is the serious biker's must-have. Top: A truly versatile fifties jacket, this version is suede.

{the wool jacket}

A tweed adaptation of the leather jacket was also extremely popular in the 1930s. It kept leather for its lining but had more details on the exterior. Its features included two-way cuffs, a shirred back, slanting pockets, convertible Cossack collars, and most important, golf tee holders, something that every jacket needs—don't you think? Some have three buttons with an additional one under the convertible collar; others have patch pockets and inverted bellows beneath the armholes, in the style of military jackets.

Toward the end of the 1930s, the combined fabric outercoat, a short Harris tweed coat in a herringbone weave with a raccoon or wombat collar and rabbit fur lining was the absolute must-have, as well as the roomy wool "lumberjack" or "mackinaw" with notched lapels, split collars to help hug the neck, and tailored sleeves.

During World War II warmth and durability were key selling points in outerwear jackets. Manufacturers were quick to remind retailers that with the imminent oil shortage, there would be a couple of long winter months ahead, hence the opportunity to sell many more "body-warming garments" such as sport vests with knit-

A houndstooth "hacking jacket" from the forties turns any man into a bit of a sport.

the eisenhower jacket

The blouse-type waist-length Eisenhower jacket was very popular in the 1950s. With set-in sleeves, slanting pockets, belted waist and zipper closure, the military-style garment was a knock-off of the British jacket envied by Ike's soldiers. Many of today's top designers (think Salvatore Ferragamo and Prada) continue to pay homage to the jacket by resurrecting it on the runways, replacing some of the wool with leather, and mix- 'n-matching it with narrow pants and long-sleeved crewnecks.

ted backs; waist-length and poplin-lined jackets with windproof knit wristlets and bottoms; and water-repellent gabardine long jackets with alpaca-like shawl collars and linings. Corduroy fingertip-length coats, especially those from the 1940s, are still pretty easy to find on the vintage market. With raglan shoulders, big pockets and railroad stitching around the hem, the coat exudes country-casual charm when worn with herringbone pants and a polo shirt. Military influence was also noted in cotton, belted, waist-length jackets with big chest pockets.

Toward the end of the forties, bold patterns and colors took over the "surcoat," an in-between-length coat that falls just above the knee. Inspired by a tunic-like garment worn over a suit of armor, it has a zipper front, an all-around belt, and saddle pockets and is a sort of precursor to the car coat. Very classic and very versatile, it can be worn with just about any style of pants—from wool gabardine or gray flannel to jeans. The end

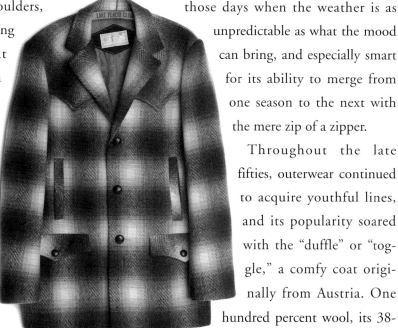

A classic example of a 1950s western-style wool plaid jacket, by Trego. See front detail, next page.

of the decade also saw the advent of the three-way short coat—still very much around and in demand today—a fur-collared outerwear jacket with a removable wool lining. "Three-way" because both the outer and inner shell can be worn separately, or together. Very practical for those days when the weather is as unpredictable as what the mood can bring, and especially smart for its ability to merge from one season to the next with the mere zip of a zipper.

Throughout the late fifties, outerwear continued to acquire youthful lines, and its popularity soared with the "duffle" or "toggle," a comfy coat originally from Austria. One hundred percent wool, its 38-inch long fleecy cloth has a hood and two huge patch pockets, and the coat/jacket closes with rope loops and wooden pegs. The double-breasted navy blue peacoat, too, a take-off on the naval uniform coat with its three or four sets of plastic black buttons with anchors on them, remains a much-relished piece from the

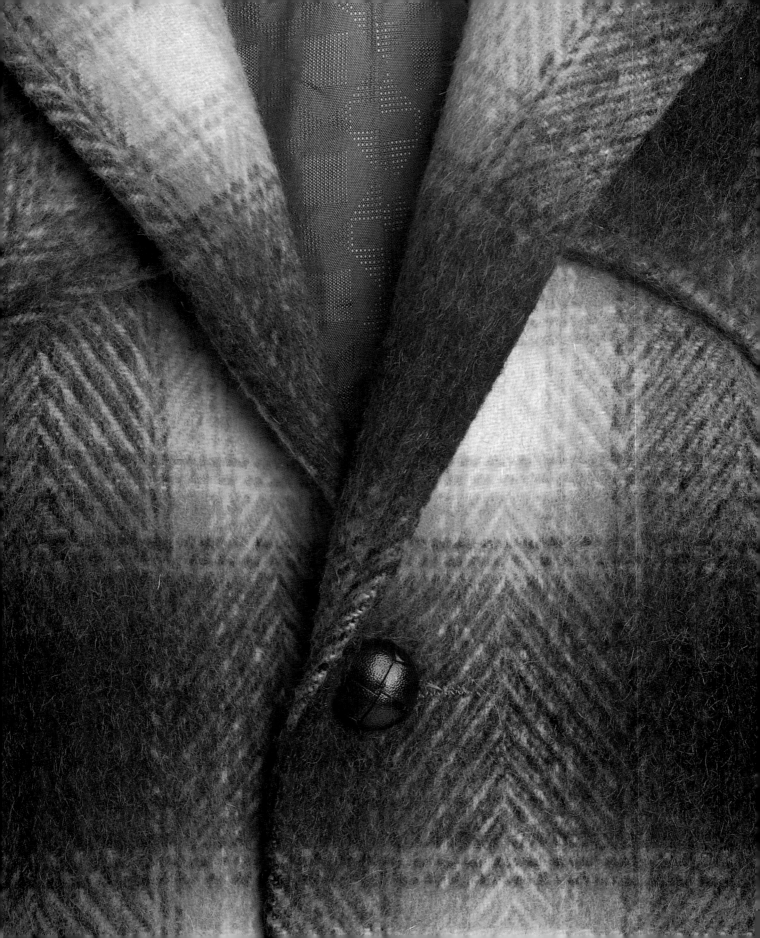

same era. With a cream cable knit turtleneck, classic khakis or jeans, the peacoat is another of today's outerwear wardrobe staples.

The sixties gave rise to a whole line of sporty outerwear, inspired from different activities like skiing, skeet shooting, and driving. This new breed, called the "commuter" or "suburbanite" by some, can be dressed up or down for fall or winter weather. The sheen rayon-and-wool gabardine short outercoat, adapted from the British shooting coat, is a very dapper option, lined in pile fabric with quilted rayon sleeves. The fabulous safari coat in a polyester-pima cotton blend is a true find. The diamond-patterned zipper jacket with vertical pockets and knitted wool collar defies taste and style. And the corduroy above-the-knee length outercoat—designed for spectator sports on campus or at stadiums—has just the right touch of rugged appeal with a deep heavy-knit wool collar, buttoned-tab side vents, leather buttons, and a tartan lining.

color classifications

According to a 1956 issue of Esquire, *there are three color classifications for jackets. These are:*

Soft tones: Grays, blues, tans, and greens.

Bright tones: With vivid accents such as red with gray, bright yellow, green or others, either alone or in combination with a neutralizing shade.

Deep tones: Browns, blacks, and deep grays and blues.

One thing to note about color is the use of sharp contrasts. For example, navy blue with white trim, turquoise with black, very dark brown with beige.

Also note that "the inside of the jacket is just as important from the fashion point of view as the outer appearance. Lustrous satin of manmade fibers is used freely in bright shades either to harmonize or contrast with the color" of the jacket.[21]

{coats}

There's no such thing as having too many coats. And by going the vintage route, you can really explore the possibilities and play around with different styles and fabrics—brushed wool fleece sports coats, tweed fly-front overcoats, camel hair polo coats—and still have enough cash left over for the fedora.

The Trench

Boasting such wearers as Winston Churchill, the Prince of Wales, George Bernard Shaw, and George Bush—without forgetting, of course, a Burberry-clad Humphrey Bogart wooing women in *Casablanca*, Gary Cooper in *Today We Live*, George C. Scott commanding his troops in *Patton*, and Michael Douglas ruling in one on *Wall Street*—the trench coat's distinctive and elegant look makes it by far the vintage coat of choice. Make sure all the accoutrements are there: wrist-straps, epaulettes, storm flap, shaped belt rings, etc. (see below). Dress it up (over a glen plaid suit and tie), dress it down (with jeans and a cotton crewneck), warm (with corduroys and a turtleneck), or cool (with lightweight khakis and a T-shirt). Either way, the classic trench will fit you and your lifestyle to a T.

totally en-trenched: a history of the "casablanca classic"

In the 1870s, London native Robert Burberry invented gabardine, a cool, lightweight, comfortable and waterproof fabric that became the material par excellence for the discerning outdoor sportsman. It wasn't until the Boer War in 1901, though, that the Burberry went into battle, proving its worth and becoming associated with deeds of valor and chivalry. All day long, officers in battle could keep cool, dry, and warm underneath the dapper cloth. It was Lord Kitchener, the commander in chief of British forces in World War I who reportedly died in a trench, however, who turned the classic Burberry double-breasted overcoat into the trench coat we know today. He had epaulettes added to the shoulder to hold binoculars, wrist-straps added to hold grenades, shaped rings on the belt for a water bottle, a storm flap at the shoulder for protection from rifle recoil, and a deep vent in the back to allow its wearer to sit on a horse in comfort. Today, no gabardine coat is deemed authentic without all this intricate symbolism.

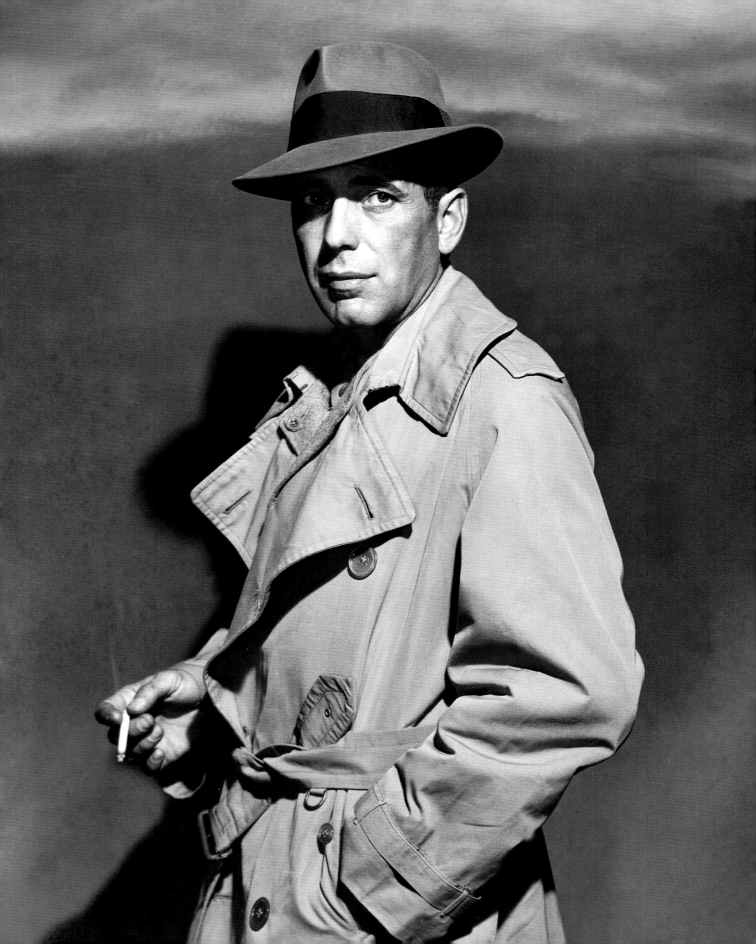

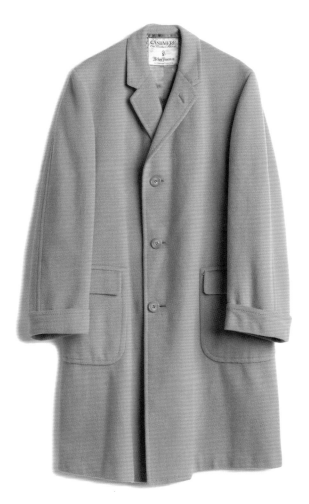

The classic camel hair coat, this one from the fifties, remains a popular outerwear staple, possibly because it is toasty warm yet lightweight.

Chesterfields, Box Coats, Fly-Front Overcoats, and Camel Hair Coats

The influence of World War I in the world of fashion is nowhere more apparent than in the form-fitting, military-style coats of the twenties and thirties. These single-breasted, narrow-shouldered numbers are trim and lightweight, they have a fly front and wide-peaked lapels, and a sewn-in belt around a high waist. Although extremely flattering on tall, lanky builds, they're not particularly well-suited for portlier men, on whom single-breasted box coats with broad shoulders work far better. The waist-defining chesterfield with long, double-breasted lapels held by a link button and extending down to the waistline, was also a big favorite among the fashion elite, especially in gray, black, dark brown, brown-and-white herringbone, and dark blue, a color often described by fashion-setters of the time as the most becoming, smartest, and richest-looking color for overgarments.

Guard Coats, Reversible Coats, Wraparounds, and Town Ulsters

These long coats, popular in the thirties and early forties, are generously cut and loosely worn, appealing to just about every man and fitting almost every stature. The dark blue guard coat, inspired by the uniform coat of the British Grenadier Guards from World War I, was an instant success when it landed on American soil in the early thirties. The loose-fitting, double-breasted coat with an inverted pleat in the back running all the way up between the shoulder blades to the collar was popular in dark blue chinchilla for winter, and dark blue, lighter weight, cheviot for spring. It makes a stunning addition to today's wardrobe.

A few years later, the reversible coat—tweed on one side, leather on the other—becomes the coat of choice. Dubbed the "Harris Tweed," it's a favorite among the college crowd and alumni alike. Its boxy silhouette attracts a wide variety of body types, and gracefully fits into any lifestyle— from a relaxed day in the country to a slick, leather-side-out night on the town.

So, too, does the "wraparound," a unique buttonless topcoat originating from England. In the mid-thirties, the loose-fitting, roomy wrap model based on traditional bathrobe design was consid-

...and the award for coat of the year goes to...

In 1928, Men's Wear *voted the chesterfield, the fly-front overcoat, the camel hair, and the box coat the four most popular styles in men's outerwear fashion, declaring them "must-haves" for every Tom, Dick, and Harry in search of some warmth, style, and comfort for the winter. Here's why:*

The Chesterfield: "This style of coat, which has for many years been a favorite with well-dressed men both here and abroad, goes hand in hand with the current derby vogue, and is a popular style with both business-men and university men this fall for day and for evening wear."

The Shapely Fly-Front: "This particular style of coat, of English origin, is quite a favorite with men who wear the single-breasted peaked lapel jacket suit. It is preferable in the tweed fabrics of the darker shades and is much in evidence at fashionable places."

The Camel Hair: "By sheer force of fashion appeal, this coat has become a favorite in the wardrobe of many thousands of well dressed men. Though it predominates in the natural camel's hair color, darker shades and patterned effects are now being introduced."

The Fly-Front Box Coat: "This is one of the most popular styles with well dressed university men. It is rather loose and straight hanging, and is usually made in tweeds and fleeces, including the entire range of the more acceptable colors. In its correct length it is 46 to 48 inches long."[22]

ered the ideal coat for driving around and lounging about. Made from camel hair or a fleece-type fabric interwoven with llama hairs, it's comfortable, warm, and easy-fitting. You can still find a few of these well-proportioned coats at your local flea or vintage shop. Some have three belt loops and pleats to add fullness below the waistline; others have side pleats from the shoulders to the belt; and others have an inverted back pleat that extends from in-between the shoulders to the waist. The wraparound is worn with the collar turned up and the belt loosely tied bathrobe-style for a casual, almost careless, and coyly disheveled look.

The town ulster is another leader in the trend toward thirties' oversized coats. Double-breasted with broad shoulders, wide lapels, four pairs of leather-covered buttons, a breast pocket, and side pockets with flaps, it has a hint of a waistline

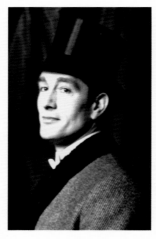

A fur collar and silk top hat spell elegance when worn with a herringbone tweed evening coat circa 1958.

while retaining a boxy, masculine shape. Woven from glen plaid, checked Harris or Shetland tweed, the coat also comes with a fur-trimmed collar—mink, opossum, or otter—for the more extravagant and fashionably daring.

The 1940s brought in a wave of shorter coats reaching only to the knees, with three sets of buttons, a rolling lapel, and rows of stitching around the bottom and at the sleeves. The length made it easy to walk around in, adding to the coat's instant popularity. It came in all sorts of fabrics and colors, with the most popular being the Harris or herringbone tweed, the blackish-brown Shetland, a blending of blue and green called "lovat green," warm browns, loam browns with gray overtones, marine blues, and tan cashmeres. Worn with a muffler, a snap-brim or pork pie hat, and thick-soled shoes, *Esquire* dubbed it "the look of self-confident taste."[23]

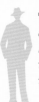

TALLY-HO! *At the 1932 United Hunts Meet in Belmont Park, Long Island, the traditional—and fashion-able—close of the New York horse racing season, hundreds of well dressed sportsmen were seen wearing broad-shouldered guard coats with shaped waist and deep folds in the back. One fashion reporter noted that "[I]n selling overcoats this season, this flash from America's racing capital might well be used to advantage in convincing a doubtful customer of the high position of this style in the world of fashion."[24]*

The tall, slender lines of men's fifties fashion gave way to pile-lined coats with plain gabardine shells. They were ideal for "bucking the crowds at the big game or battling winds on the way to the commuters' special."[25] Tweed overcoats, chesterfields in muted shades, and dark blue double-breasted cashmere polo-type coats with patch pockets and a half-belt conquered the streets. To this day, their quality is irreproachable and almost unsurpassed.

Then in the sixties, everything—including coats—took a radical turn, stepping out and away from the classic shapes of the past few decades and into a new line of outergarments. The maxi-coat in particular, something that looks like a throwback from the Napoleonic era with its high waist, brass military buttons, and long, flared bottom, became all the rage. Every single designer—from Pierre Cardin to Cerruti—made their own version with a twist, using a vari-

fur-get it!

By the early sixties, fur had become extremely popular. From natural muskrat to black curly lamb, Brazilian leopard, kangaroo, mink, alpaca, antelope, bear, giraffe- and zebra-stenciled calf, no fur was too unusual for fashion aficionados. Things got so out of hand that Congress ultimately passed a series of guidelines concerning the use of fur on clothing, as well as strict rules and regulations when it came to providing consumers with adequate labeling information. In essence, every fur selling for over $5 (in 1952) had to have, in part, the following information stated on its labels, sales slips, and ads:

"The true English name of the animal from which the fur has come...

"The name of the country of origin of all imported furs...

"The proper information as to whether the fur has been 'treated,'
e.g., bleached, dyed, tip-dyed or in any way artificially colored...

"Disclosure as to whether the garment is entirely, or even partially, composed of
paws, sides, flanks, gills, tails or waste fur..."[24]

ety of colors and fabrics like cashmere, wool, Perisan lamb, leather, and twill with lots of fur trim. Its double-breasted front, wide lapels, slanted flap pockets, deep inverted back pleat, and narrow armholes flow graciously on tall figures. (At 48 inches long, you've got to have the height to pull this one off!)

In the late sixties and early seventies, though, Americans started developing an ecological conscience. With controversy in the air, real fur began taking a back seat to fake, man-made, 100 percent artificial, imitation fur. Vintage stores are usually stocked with these babies, very popular in the seventies because they were inexpensive to manufacture, and better yet, had the look and feel of fur, minus the guilt and the price tag. Black Orlon looks just like black seal, viscose rayon dyed off-white is a dead ringer for pony skin, and silver-gray pile makes a great imitation chinchilla.

There you have it. A brief look at what's out there in the vintage outerwear department, and there truly is something for everyone, even the finickiest of dressers. So pull up your sleeves, dig your heels in deep, and jump right in. You're bound to resurface with the apple of your eye.

coat classifications

According to a 1956 issue of Esquire, *there are three basic coat classifications:*

• Waist-length coats influenced by the Eisenhower jacket (see "Jackets," page 202)

• Intermediate-length coats that measure about thirty-two inches for a man of average height, just a tad longer than conventional business suit jackets.

• Thirty-five to thirty-six-inch length coats, described as four-button "suburbans." Many are reversible, with soft, fleece-like fabric on one side and water-repellent fabric on the other.[27]

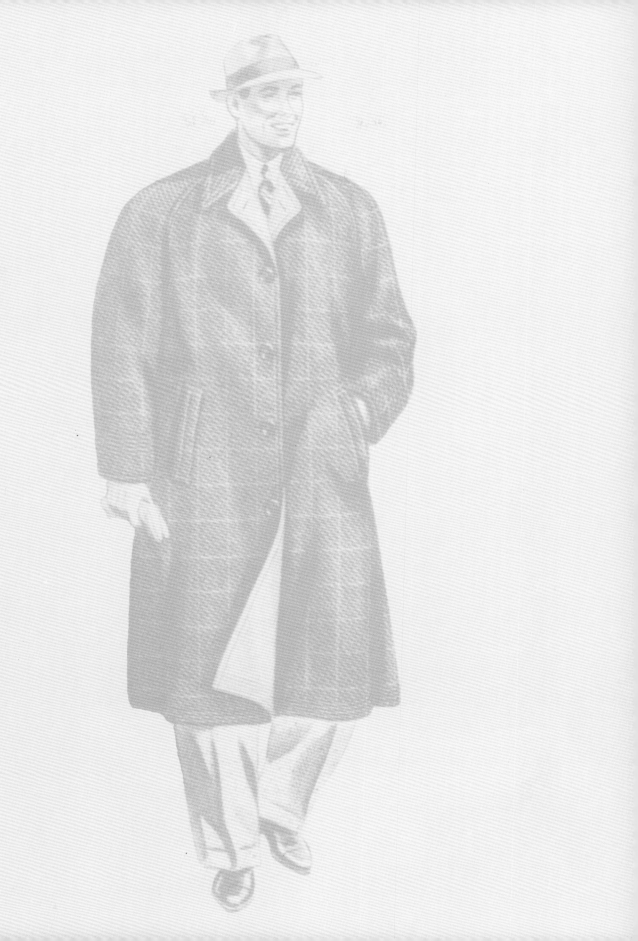

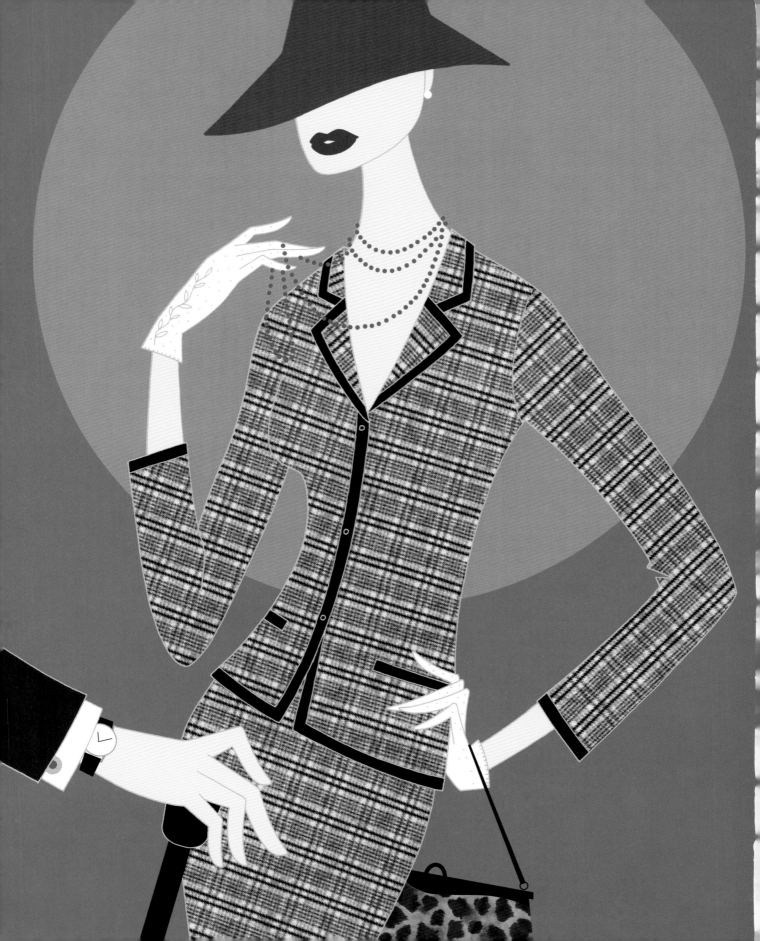

{8}

accessories

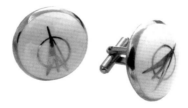

"Elegance is innate.
It has nothing to do with being well-dressed."

—*Diana Vreeland*

family jewels

When you talk to seasoned vintage shoppers and wearers, they tend to admit that they got their feet wet buying accessories. Before plunging in with a full retro suit or gown, they went for smaller pieces, maybe a Bakelite bracelet or two, a fun tie from the 1940s, or needle-nosed cowboy boots from the 1950s—something to gradually ease them into the world of vintage.

Incorporating a few vintage accessories into your look—a leopard-print pillbox hat, a fringed piano shawl, some '70s platforms, a pair of square-framed Buddy Holly glasses, or an old fedora, for example—is the perfect way to revamp a tired wardrobe and to accentuate your individual style. It's inexpensive, fun, and a terrific outlet for creativity. Besides, it's a heck of a lot easier than buying an entire outfit. In a shopping environment that doesn't always make it easy to try things on (does the old "slipping-on-pants-under-the-skirt-behind-the-rack" trick sound familiar?), there's something to be said for surreptitiously gliding

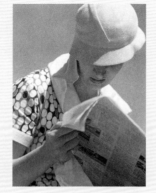

The sassiness and sex appeal of the 1920s "cloche" never goes out of style.

into a pair of mules for sizing, pinning on a rhinestone brooch at the counter to experience an instant sense of glitter, or checking out a pair of antique cufflinks or 1920s circular-framed glasses without revealing too much skin.

When it comes to shopping for vintage accessories, the ground rules are simple: don't spend too much. Chances are, most of the stuff that you'll come across in bins and boxes at consignment or secondhand stores has already been picked through for valuables. In other words, don't expect to find that one-of-a-kind Trifari pin or original Kelly bag, or that intact Tiffany watch from the 1950s. If, on the other hand, you do come across something that smells like a jackpot, feel free to ask the seller plenty of questions: How old is the piece? Who was the original owner? How was it made? Where was it made? Could there possibly be any paperwork on the piece? All of this without blowing the nature of your find, of course.

"What shoe aficionados find so appealing in vintage is the level of detail and quality of material."

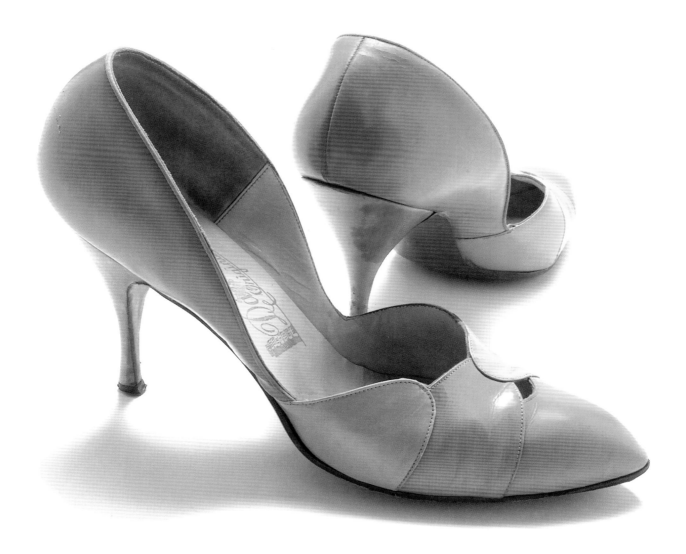

They're more comfortable than you think! In the early 1950s, the stiletto dramatically pierced its way into fashion.

{women's accessories}

"Don't underestimate the power of a little sparkle and glitter. Provoke a plunging neckline with a strategically placed vintage rhinestone brooch or necklace; add some edge to a lapel with an Art Deco pin; or bring a jingle to your step with stacked Bakelite bangles."

Move over discount outlets and sample sales! The way to purge your urge for a little treat and to satisfy that craving for something different is to dive right into the accessory bin at your favorite vintage clothing haunt. There's nothing more exhilarating than sifting through trinkets from another place and time—silky scarves, glittery purses, chunky earrings, oodles of bangles, satin opera-length gloves, tiny lipstick cases, shoes, shoes, and more shoes—in search of that perfect little treasure that you don't really need until you cast your eyes on it—and then you absolutely, positively have to have it "because you've been looking for one just like it for so long!"

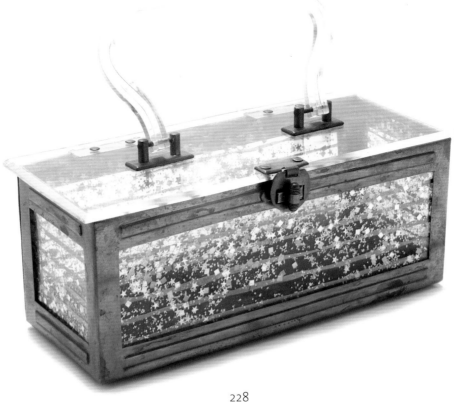

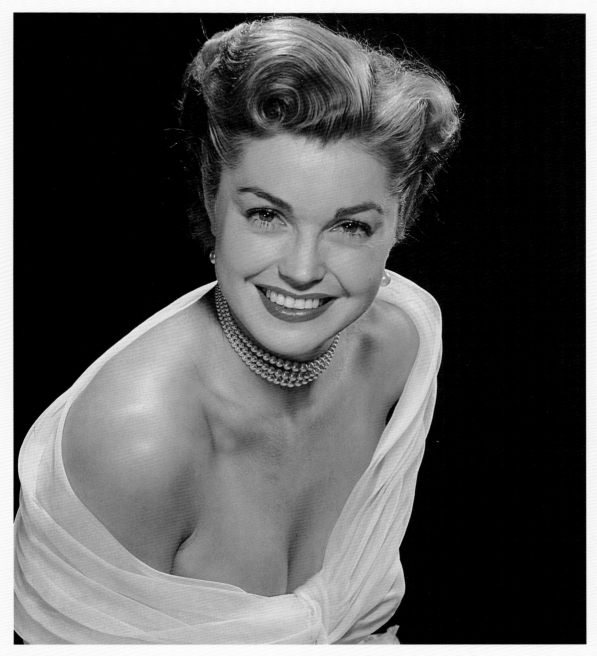

It's all in the details: The smallest accent can make a world a difference, as in this three-strand pearl choker modeled by Esther Williams, or a fabulously starry lucite handbag (opposite).

{jewelry}

Diamonds may be a girl's best friend, but no one in their right mind would ever pass up a fabulous vintage fake. Over the past few years, vintage costume jewelry—twenty-plus-year-old pieces made from non-precious materials and stones—has become so hot that certain collectibles can fetch as much as, if not more than, contemporary pieces of fine jewelry. The reason for its popularity is simple: vintage costume jewelry is unique, usually of better quality than contemporary costume jewelry, and carries with it a bit of history and personality. Some collectors argue that wearing vintage costume jewelry is like wearing a piece of art. Each piece is original and tells us about art currents, social trends, and fashions of the times.

Costume jewelry has been around since the early 1700s when "paste stones"—high-quality imitations of glass composition, imported from Venice, were used as alternatives to genuine diamonds and gemstones. But it wasn't until after World War I that costume jewelry took on an entirely different status. At that time, Parisian designers like Coco Chanel and Jean Patou began showing their clothes with fun fakes. Chanel in particular thought that women should be able to change their jewelry as often as they did their clothes, and often mixed real jewelry with costume pieces. Soon thereafter, American manufacturers like Eisenberg Ice Jewelry and Miriam Haskell quickly stepped up production. Originally, costume jewelry consisted of copies of authentic precious pieces, look-alikes meant in part to deter theft and, of course, to offer the illusion of wealth and glamour to the general public. In the late 1920s, however, designers stopped making "forgeries," focusing more on original designs made from non-precious materials, creating pieces that were bolder, brighter, and more ornate.

Most pieces made before the late '30s or early '40s were not signed because they weren't deemed important enough to bear the creator's name. The signed pieces you might be fortunate enough to come across were most likely made after that. Look for any of the following names and you'll be sure to have hit a gold mine: Hattie Carnegie, Elsa Schiaparelli, Miriam Haskell, Cinner,

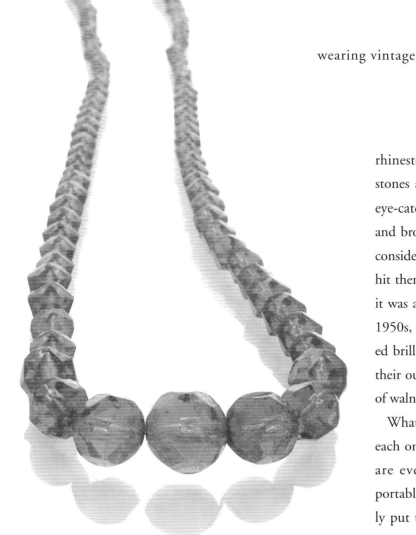

rhinestones and faux gems were hot items. Big stones and glitzy metal were combined to create eye-catching pieces such as rings, bib-necklaces, and brooches. Bakelite, a molded plastic that was considered very modern at the time, was also a big hit then (and is blazingly popular even now), and it was a less expensive alternative to metal. In the 1950s, women wore large-scale pieces that included brilliant brooches (color-coordinated to match their outfits) with chunky button earrings the size of walnuts. Charm bracelets were all the rage.

What makes charm bracelets so special is that each one carries a lifetime of history, and no two are ever alike. Some are like scrapbooks or portable time capsules, carefully and painstakingly put together over decades; others are a revelation into the soul; and others still a true declaration of love. Take the charm bracelets worn by the Duchess of Windsor: On her wedding day she wore a bracelet with jewel-studded crosses, each one bearing an inscription from her husband; another favorite of hers was a small wrist chain from which dangled a frog, a ladybug, an entwined WE, and a snippet of the duke's

Monet, Lalique, Butler & Wilson, Eisenberg, Trifari, Coro, Napier, Kenneth Jay Lane, Nettie Rosenstein, and Weiss, to name just a few.

Each decade is remembered for a particular style. In the 1920s, pearls (both real and artificial) were important accessories, and long strands of them, draped in endless ropes, graced the neck of every self-respecting flapper. Geometric shapes and streamlined designs are another telltale characteristic of this Art Deco period. In the 1930s and 1940s, jewelry made with large glittering

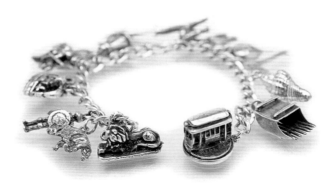

A charm bracelet can be a work-in-progress over many years, with charms added to mark such milestones as birthdays, graduation, and career moves.

hair. Then there are the little charms Prince Charles presented to Diana every year for her birthday.

Charm bracelets from the 1950s were basically divided into two categories—classic and kitsch—both still available on the vintage market today.

The classic charm bracelet in silver, gold, or gold-plated metal is the one to which individual charms were carefully added over time. Each charm was individually designed and manufactured with various precious metals, enamel, semi-precious stones, glass beads, or pearls. Some charms had moveable parts, and others did not. You can still find the more expensive bracelets on the market, already jingling with mementos from someone else's life, or you can put together your

charmed, i'm sure...

A little jingle goes a long way. Especially when it comes with a small teapot, the Eiffel Tower, a bowling pin, a graduation cap, a bite-sized shovel, a ballet slipper, a gumball machine with tiny colored beads, and a miniature shoe. Charm bracelets, and their soft music that precedes a wearer's entrance, have been casting spells on generations for ages. Credit most likely goes to Queen Victoria in the 1890s, when she wore their precursor, a small chain bracelet from which dangled lockets containing family portraits. Fast-forward some sixty-odd years and one continent over, and you find young American women in the 1950s buying plain chain bracelets and hooking on charms as mementos of events in their lives (first prom, first kiss, graduation, birthday, summer trip, engagement, marriage, birth, anniversary, etc.) or of places to which they have been.

bakelite or bust

If you're not sure whether the fabulous set of bangles you've just picked up are the real McCoy or not, you might want to try one of these Bakelite-busting tests:

The "clunk" test: Because Bakelite is heavier than most plastics, pieces should clunk, not click, together.

The smell test: Dealers suggest rubbing the piece. Real Bakelite gives off a slight formaldehyde odor. Or, if you coincidentally happen to be near running hot water, dip an edge of the piece under water for about 30 seconds, then smell it. When wet, Bakelite has a distinctive, almost acidic, odor.

The Formula 409 test: Dip a cotton swab into the liquid, and dab a small area on the back of the piece. If the material is Bakelite and it hasn't been refinished, the swab will now have a dark yellow stain on it. Make sure you thoroughly rinse the piece afterwards, then worry about getting escorted out of the flea market. [28]

own bits of history by picking out individual charms throughout your vintage travels, and hooking them onto a favorite bracelet, chain, or belt.

The kitschier charm bracelet, on the other hand, was more of a novelty item than a piece of jewelry. Made from plastic or cheap metal such as tin or aluminum, the bracelet was sold with all its charms already on, for an immediate jingling effect. Today, you can potentially haggle one of these bracelets down to about $15–$20. Not a bad investment for a million-dollar conversation piece.

Pieces from the 1960s were made to match the revolutionary fabrics and materials used in fashion. Metal, Lucite, and Bakelite jewelry complemented Space Age design: chunky rings and watches with clear bands, metal mesh bracelets and "flower power" necklaces with oversized beads.

Dubbed by jewelry experts and vintage aficionados as "the antidepressant of the accessory world" because of its inherent mood-lifting qualities, Bakelite jewelry—bangles, brooches, earrings, and necklaces—is downright addictive. Once you've purchased your first bit of brightly-hued translucent wonder, you'll join the ranks of avid Bakelite collectors. The colorful pieces, exquisite on their own yet to die for when worn in clusters, are made from heavy plastic—thermosetting phenolic formaldehyde resin, to be more precise. The sturdy material was patented in 1909 by chemist Leo H. Baekland, who created it primarily for industrial use. It wasn't until

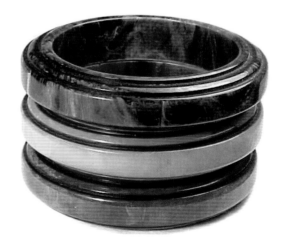

the 1920s that jewelry designers started to pick up on the appeal of Bakelite as a medium with which to create fun and relatively inexpensive creations. With experimentation, more and more colors became available, and in the 1940s and '50s, Bakelite anything—including radios, telephones, and bowling balls—was de rigueur.

Because few Bakelite pieces were ever signed or dated, it's hard to tell exactly how old they are. Collectors will agree, however, that it is safe to assume that most Bakelite was made between 1920 and 1950. And if you find a piece with "star dust," tiny bits of metallic glitter suspended in the Bakelite itself, chances are you're holding something from 1936 or 1937, the only time "star dust" was used. Another tell-tale sign of age and authenticity, especially when it comes to pins or pieces with claps, is the hardware itself: It should be riveted or set directly into the Bakelite. Any piece where the hardware is glued on is most likely to have been made after 1949.

Although Bakelite is a type of plastic, it is not just any ordinary type of plastic. It's heavier than most plastics, and just doesn't feel like plastic. Anyone who has heard the distinctive "clunk" of Bakelite bangles rapping together knows that a "clunk" is a far cry from a regular plastic "click." The soft, translucent resin is also one that can break and age, albeit gracefully. In fact, like fine wine, it oxidizes with time, which means that it changes color and becomes more dense and mellow. Pieces that were once bright pink or tomato red have turned into rich browns; intense blues soften up and turn olive green; clears develop an apple-juice tint; and whites go cream. Look for pieces that have clever patterns and unusual, Deco-inspired designs. Some even have moving parts like branches with dangling fruit or windmills that move. Wear them with everything from bathing suits to evening wear. Elegance dresses up as well as down.

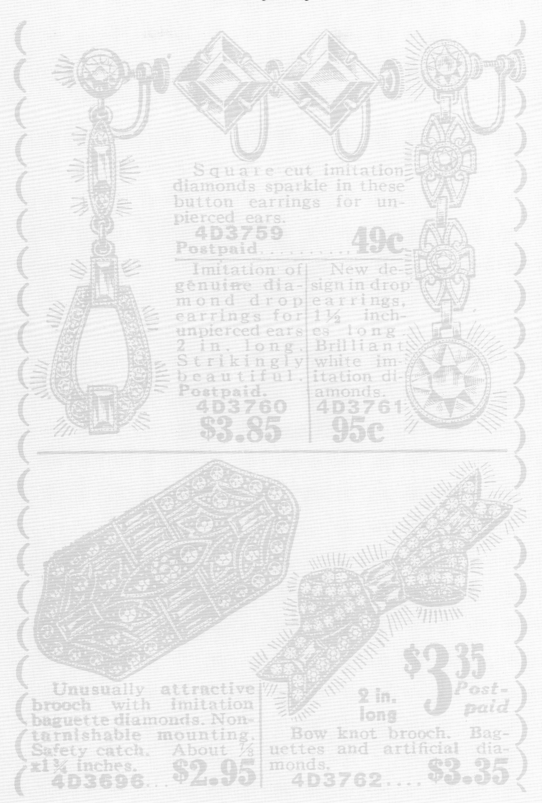

Square cut imitation diamonds sparkle in these button earrings for un-pierced ears.
4D3759
Postpaid.......... **49c**

Imitation of genuine dia-mond drop earrings for unpierced ears 2 in. long. Strikingly beautiful. Postpaid.
4D3760
$3.85

New de-sign in drop earrings, 1½ inch-es long. Brilliant white im-itation di-amonds.
4D3761
95c

Unusually attractive brooch with imitation baguette diamonds. Non-tarnishable mounting. Safety catch. About ⅞ x1¾ inches.
4D3696... **$2.95**

Bow knot brooch. Bag-uettes and artificial dia-monds.
4D3762.... **$3.35**

2 in. long **$3³⁵** Post-paid

{shoes}

Whether it's pointy-toe pumps from the '50s, clear vinyl sandals from the '60s, or a full-fledged platform from the '70s, what shoe aficionados find so appealing in vintage footwear is the level of detail and the quality of material, virtually impossible to replicate on contemporary counterparts without sending their price sky-high: hand-sewn seams and heels that are nailed in, not glued on; beads and sequins that are sewn in, not pasted; fabric- or leather-covered buttons and buckles; heels decorated with hand embroidery; and mules adorned with real feathers and rows of rhinestones.

The key thing to remember when shopping for vintage footwear is to try it on. Shoe sizes from the '30s or '50s are not the same as they are today; European sizes are different from American, and shoes often take on a wearer's imprint that might not match your own. It's important that the shoe fits comfortably in the store, as there is little chance that it can be "broken in" or stretched out later.

The 1950s: European curves

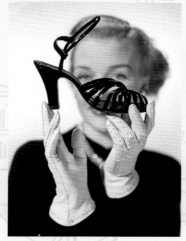

Stacked to perfection, a strappy sandal from the 1950s could be fresh from the pages of today's Vogue.

styles of the times

The 1940s: Femininity and elegance were redefined, as styles softened, soles lightened, and platform edges rounded. Brightly colored leathers, big straps, and buttons adorned shoes. Chunky cork bottoms were introduced to America by designer Salvatore Ferragamo, as well as his "invisible sandal" with uppers of nylon threads. The tapered heel also made its debut, and it was covered in everything from satin to delicate hand embroidery.

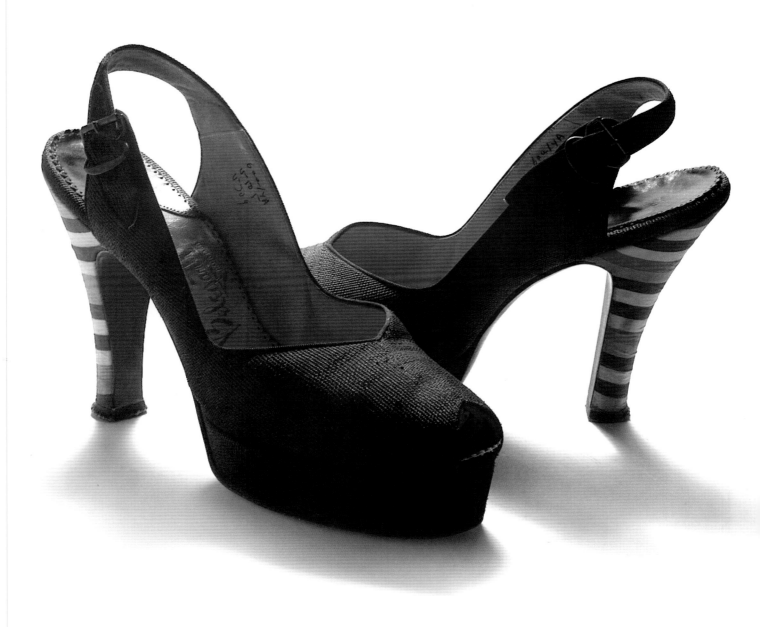

Rounded edges were characteristic of forties shoes,
as with this pair of open-toe platform slingbacks by Belaganti.

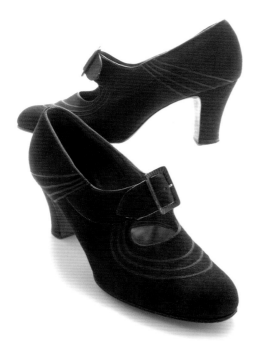

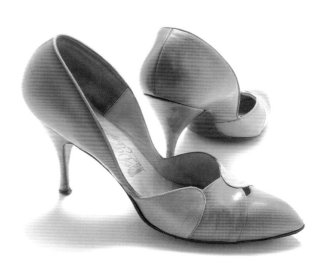

This parade of footwear is a shoe-lover's dream-come-true—and they are all vintage finds! From elegant thirties suede with soft leather bottoms (upper left) to rainbow slip-ons circa 1970 (bottom right) via the quintessential Mod go-go boots from the sixties and a toothsome array of sandals and spectators, there's a shoe to fit every fancy.

gave way to angular forms. Toes narrowed; stilettos and "spikes"—heels made from metal spikes embedded in plastic—dramatically pierced their way into fashion. Redefining the foot as the new erogenous zone, the slick, narrow heel epitomized '50s glamour-girl style. Although they proved to be hazardous to the female foot and were banned from certain public places because of the divots they would leave on floor surfaces, stilettos remained immensely popular, with gold spikes, leopard skin, and brocade favorites on the dance floor.

The 1960s: As constricting styles loosened up, the heel lost some height and a new emphasis on

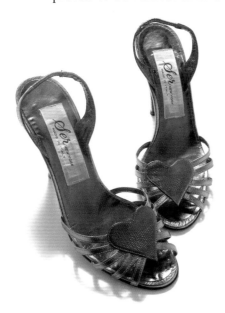

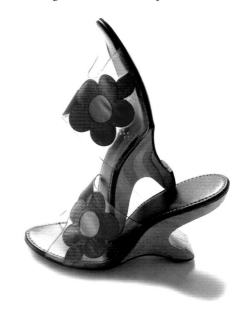

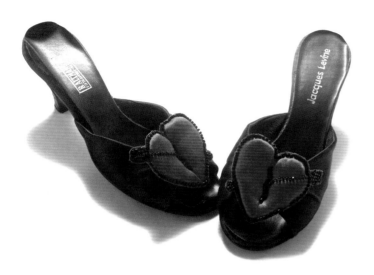

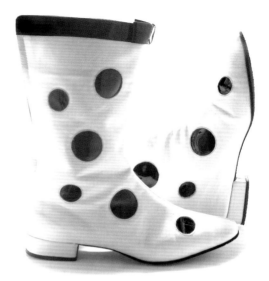

geometry took over footwear fashion. Shiny patent leathers, plastics, and metallic-finished leathers were used to reflect the new Space Age chic popularized by Pierre Cardin.

The 1970s: The platform stole the fashion stage. Cork was resurrected from the 1930s and 1940s and used to create fabulously fun footwear, with shoes, boots, or sandals sometimes as high as ten inches off the ground! While some platforms remained simple and unadorned, others made ideal canvases for everything from detailed painting to intricate beading, embroidery, and sculpting. One pair was even designed like a small aquarium in which a live goldfish was meant to swim around, although one can't speculate as to how long the creature actually survived a vigorous evening at the disco. Some platforms were adorned with plastic fruit and leaves, others were transformed into stacked heels and wedged soles.

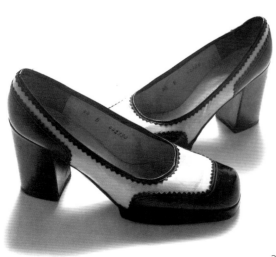

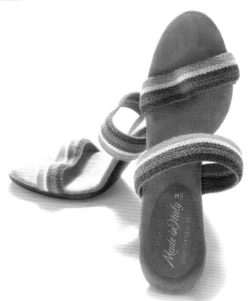

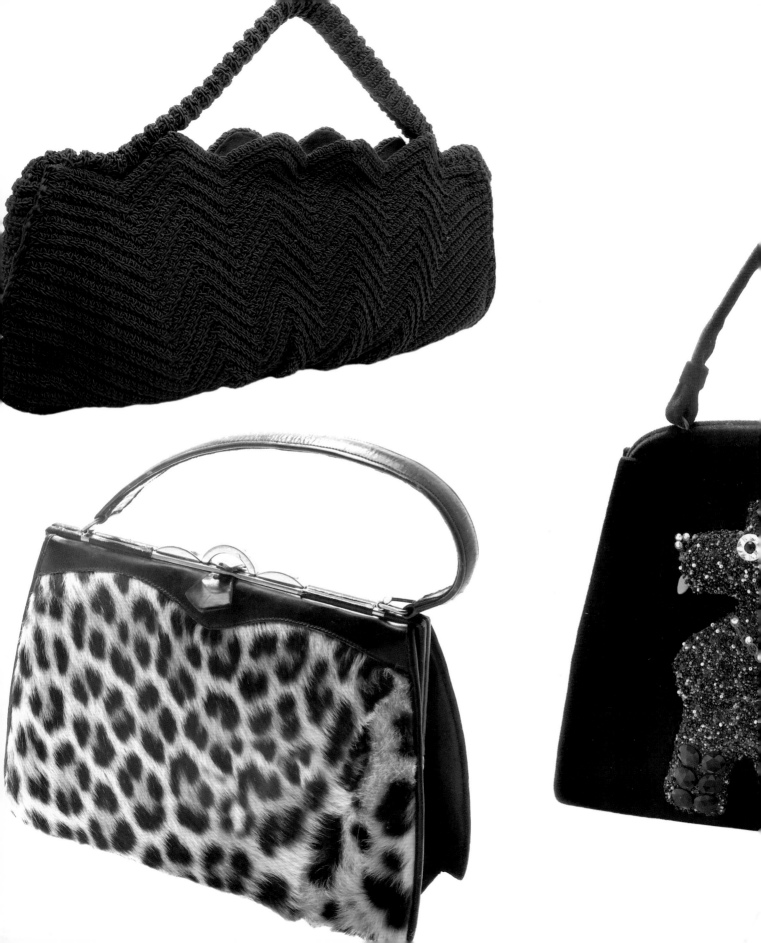

Variations in vintage: Whether beaded (1940s), French poodled (1950s), leopard spotted (1960s), embroidered, sequined or faux croc (1970s), there's a purse to complete every outfit—and suit every mood.

During your vintage forays, keep your eyes peeled for Enid Collins creations. These unusual and over-the-top bags are very evocative of the whimsical fashion styles of the '60s and the '70s. Some are covered with faux jewels or fabric; others, known as "box bags" are made from decorated wood and have short handles. Also look for minaudières, those small hard-cased evening clutches de-signed to hold only the essentials. They often come in unusual shapes like that of a bird, a cat, and owl's head, or an egg. Jeweler Alfred Van Cleef (as in Van Cleef and Arpels) was rumored to have coined the term "minaudière," which comes from the French for "coquettish air," when he saw Florence Gould, the wealthy wife of a railroad baron, using a cigarette tin to hold her precious few belongings. The bite-size jewels were originally made from precious metal, and they were adorned with precious or semi-precious stones. Since then, minaudières have been made in all sorts of hard materials, including plastic, aluminum, and ivory. They are ideal for an evening out, when all you need is something to hold your lipstick, a key, and a folded bill.

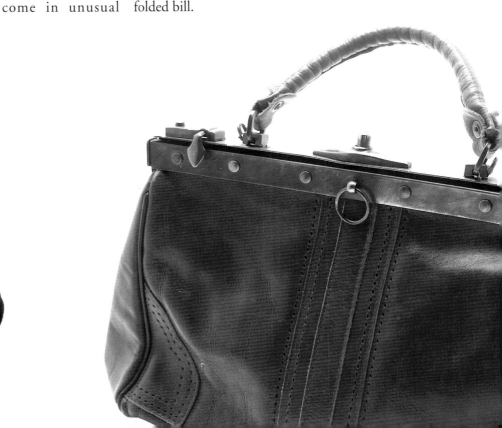

{hats, belts & gloves}

When you're rummaging through accessory bins or looking at cases of miscellaneous "stuff," it's easy to get overwhelmed by the sheer volume and variety, especially after a full day of shopping. One trick to keep in mind (and to keep your head from spinning), is to mentally break down what you're looking at into distinct categories. You don't want to be dazed by a mass of treasures; instead, you want to be looking at sunglasses, scarves, hats, gloves, and belts, separately. If the items are not clearly divided up or visibly marked in the display, train your eye to scan over all the pairs of sunglasses first, then move on to something else. While you focus on one category at a time, you'll have a better idea of what you're looking for and what most strikes your fancy. Also remember that the originality of certain pieces can get lost in the shuffle when there are so many other distractions about. Since accessories are easy to try on, don't hesitate to ask for something to be removed from a case or pulled

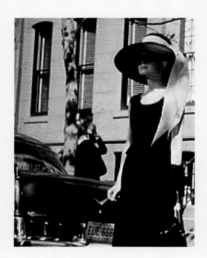

Audrey Hepburn in her signature wide-brimmed hat as Holly Golightly in Breakfast at Tiffany's.

off a mannequin so that you can appreciate it on its own. When sifting though bins of scarves, pull them out individually and play with them for a while.

Scarves, for example, are a very easy and inexpensive way of adding style and color to any outfit, and effectively dressing up business attire to ease it into evening. Loosely tie a silk square around your neck and tuck it neatly inside a jacket. Wrap one elegantly over your head and knot it casually under the chin for an incognito walk down the street, or drape a shawl around your shoulders to fight off a little chill in the air when a jacket or sweater is too much. Tighten one around your waist as a makeshift belt, or wrap a fringed and embroidered piano shawl from the thirties around your hips for a body-hugging skirt with lots of character. Remember, too, that slightly damaged or stained scarves can be used around the house as a way to dress up a table or soften the edges of a dresser top.

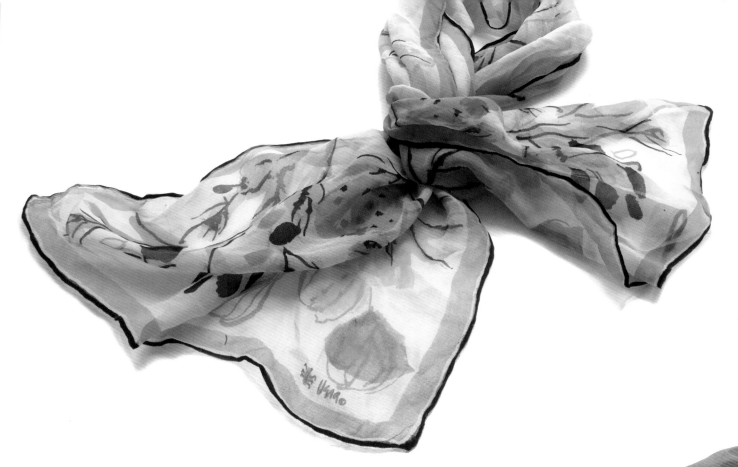

Authentic Emilio Pucci, Vera, and Hermès scarves always bear the designer's signature, like these original silk squares from the sixties.

You can even create "mood lighting" by draping one over a lampshade. Bandanas, which you can sometimes snatch up for as little as fifty cents apiece, make great napkins!

Scarves come in a variety of shapes, sizes, and colors. There are squares, rectangles, bandanas, mufflers, pocket squares, wraps, and shawls, to name just a few. Made from silk, nylon, cotton, wool, or any variation thereof, they can be hand-painted, silk-screened, printed, or have patterns woven right into the fabric. The highest quality scarves tend to be made from ultra heavy silk, featuring such household names as Hermès and Gucci. These scarves are screen printed, a technique in which each color is individually printed on the scarf. The more complicated and colorful

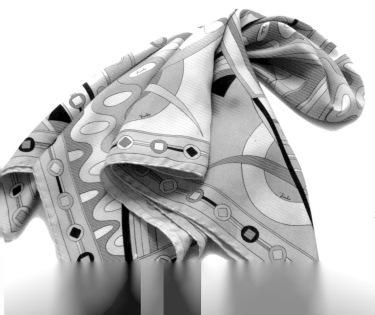

245

{accessories}

{men's accessories}

"From timepieces to top hats, men's vintage accessories, or "furnishings," carry a special cachet, an original flair that is seldom replicated in contemporary merchandise."

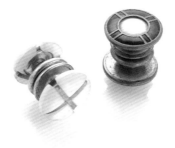

What man could possibly resist a tie from the 1950s, hand-painted with palm trees or geometric designs? Or a pair of perfectly worn-in, "blister-free," Tony Lama boots from the 1970s? Or Art Deco sterling and onyx cufflinks from the 1940s, perfectly designed to team up with a brand-new tuxedo shirt? Not many, which is why the men's vintage accessory market has become every bit as popular as the women's.

A hint of a cufflink (like the Art Deco pair pictured here), a hand-painted tie from the forties, or a stylish fedora is all you need to jump start your wardrobe.

From timepieces to top hats, men's vintage accessories, or "furnishings," carry a special cachet, an original flair that is seldom replicated in contemporary merchandise. And because vintage accessories tend to be more accessible from a financial standpoint, you can indulge in a variety of designs and special accoutrements, and still have enough left over for a nightcap after the opera.

must-have vintage treasure trinkets

Chains, wristwatches, pocket watches, eyeglasses and sunglasses, eyeglass cases, cufflinks, neckties, tie tacks, tie bars, tie pins, lapel pins, gloves, ascots, belts, vest chains, cummerbunds, stud sets, buckles, socks, rings, key chains, wallets, money clips, shoes, umbrellas, hats, cigar cases, and bowties.

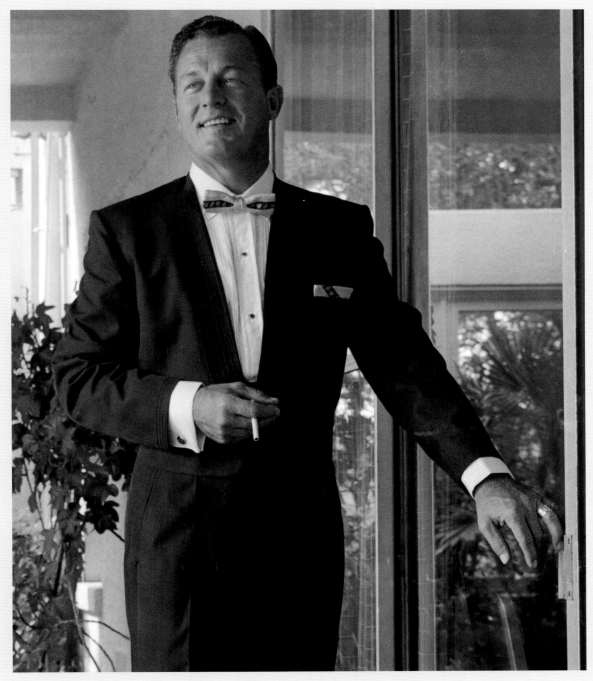

Cufflinks, studs, a bow tie, and a pocket square...
these essential accessories complete the look of this 1955 tuxedo.

{neckties}

Vintage ties are always fun to shop for. In vivid colors and patterns, they're more decorative than most contemporary ones, adding character and flavor to virtually any shirt. Vintage ties start at about $5 each, which means that you can treat yourself to a handful—one for every day of the week—for less than what it costs to buy a new one. Or, if you're on a lucky streak, you can splurge on one of the few designed and signed by the surrealist artist Salvador Dali during his stay in California in the 1940s, or a nice silk one that bears the Elsa Schiaparelli or Countess Mara signature.

Ranging from the wide, flashy ties of the '40s to the skinny rockabilly ones of the early '60s, there is a tie for every suit, shirt, and mood. The most prized vintage ties are hand-painted on silk or hand-block-printed on rayon, depicting a variety of designs, including dogs, horses, abstract designs, bathing beauties, golfers, or Western motifs. And while you're at the tie bin, keep your eyes peeled for fringed silk and rayon scarves and ascots from the 1940s. They look superb tucked into a dark overcoat or draped over a dinner jacket.

The origins of the tie can be traced back to the "cravat," a distinctive cloth or ribbon worn around the neck for identification purposes, and knotted at the front to make sure it didn't come off. It was worn by Roman legionnaires on the battlefield, and by Croatian mercenaries who served under Louis XIV. Adapted by French aristocrats, the cravat was briefly dismissed during the French Revolution, only to regain popularity shortly thereafter.

Throughout the centuries, the necktie hasn't changed much in shape, except to adapt to decreasing size and stiffness of shirt collars. Although simple in appearance, the necktie actually requires fine craftsmanship. It consists of four separate pieces of cloth, each one carefully measured and cut on the bias to prevent twisting when the tie is knotted. To ensure a proper knot that holds, the tie's inner seam is slip-stitched and left loose on the thin end of the tie.

Going the vintage route for bowties and neckties is the obvious choice, especially if selection, originality, and style are what you're after. Opposite: Fifties ties are so decorative, you can frame the one's you don't wear!

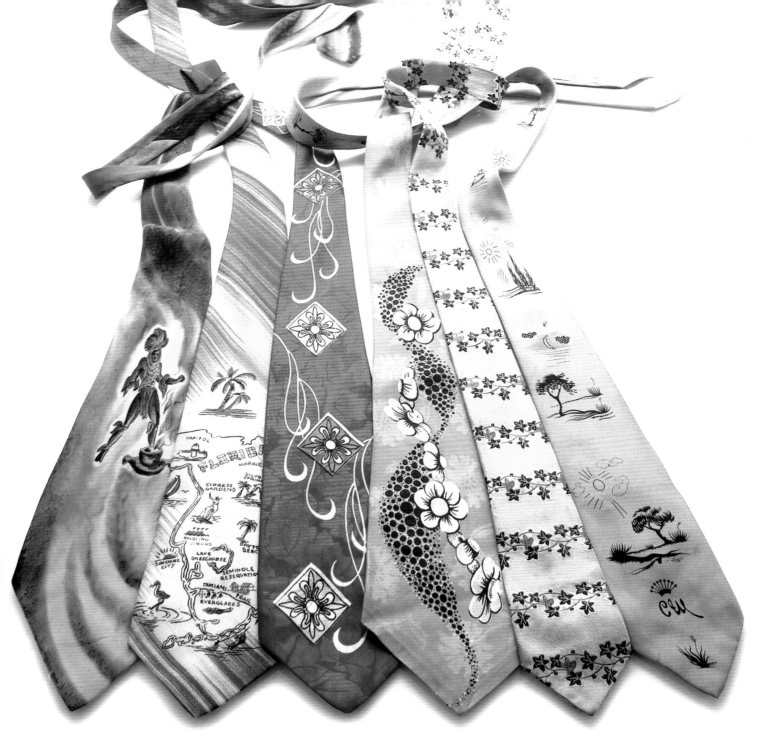

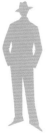 **TYING ONE ON** *The tie is one of the few articles of male clothing that doesn't have much practical purpose, if any, yet continues, relentlessly, to be a fashion staple at the office, at formal functions, and at social gatherings for a touch of color and elegance. And while that little piece of fabric appears to be purely decorative, some men seem to take longer choosing a tie than they do the rest of the outfit. The tie is the one clothing item that allows him to "cut loose," to express himself—because even the most conservative suit is well mated with a flamboyant silk tie.*

{footwear}

You don't have to be a swing dancer or own a zoot suit to appreciate the beauty of a pair of two-toned, squared-toed spectators or leather wing tips. Although the original designs were worn with wide-legged pinstriped pants, they look positively fabulous when paired with jeans, pleated linens, or cuffed gabardines. Notice the quality of the leather, the sturdiness of the soles and the intricate detailing. Avoid leather that is cracked (it will only get worse with wear), and check for worn heels or holes in the soles. Always try on shoes at the store and don't rely on sizing: a size eleven from the 1950s doesn't necessarily correspond to a size eleven today, and European

if the shoe fits...

• Scientists estimate that the first foot covering dates back to the Ice Age, 5,000,000 years ago. It consisted of a piece of rawhide fastened to the foot with a tendon.

• The "tab" or "teb" was an early Egyptian sandal made from plaited papyrus leaves.

• The Roman Campagus, a lace-up military sandal, indicated a soldier's rank. The higher the sandal, the higher the rank.

• In medieval times, shoes were sometimes so pointy and long that they were difficult and dangerous to walk in, and laws were enacted to limit their pointiness.

• Long-toed shoes like the klomp, the poulaine, and the crackow were popular styles in fourteenth-century England.

• Platforms made their first appearance in the fifteeth-century.

• Buckles were invented in the sixteenth-century; laces were invented in 1790.

• The first Oxford appeared between 1665 and 1670. It was a heavy leather boot worn by seventeenth-century Oxford University students.

• The standard shoe sizes we use today were developed in 1792.

• Up until the 1850s, shoes were made on straight shoe forms (lasts), which meant that there was no difference between the right and left foot

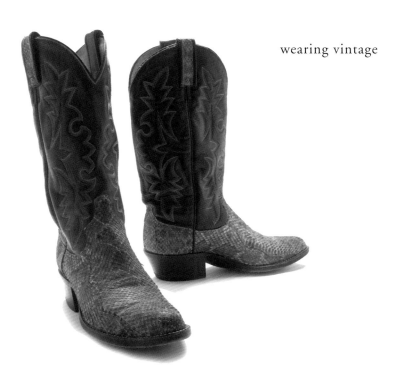

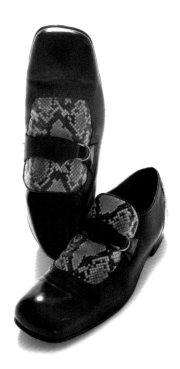

Say it with snakeskin; whether you are donning fabulous fifties cowboy boots or adorable 1960s oxfords.

sizes and lasts differ from American ones. Also look for cap toe shoes, saddle oxfords, and shoes with lizard or mesh fronts.

Cowboy boots are another popular item on the vintage footwear front. Wearers of Western-wear swear by them as a way to bypass the initial discomfort factor usually associated with brand new boots. In other words, you don't have to deal with breaking them in. And boot manufacturers tend to agree: older models were better made. They were constructed with hard, leather-capped toes to protect feet from horse hooves, as opposed to the cheaper plastic nylon-formed cap toes used today. The quality of the leather was superior, sometimes yielding to more exotic skins like python, anteater, and kangaroo (a popular skin in the 1950s before the endangered species law took effect in the U.S.).

According to boot makers, the first cowboy boots were made around the early 1800s. They were squared off at the toe and had a fairly low heel. A more rounded toe showed up about thirty years later, followed by the pointed—or needle-nosed—toe popular in the 1950s. Although black boots with pointed toes and low-slung heels remain the most popular style, whip-stitched styles from the 1950s, Tony Lama lizard boots from the 1960s, and square-toe boots from the 1940s through the 1970s featuring colorful novelty inlays like cacti and wildflowers are increasingly in demand.

Brands to look for are Justin (established in 1879), Tony Lama, Lucchese, Acme Boots, Stallion, and Laredo.

{treatment for your treasures}

Whether you've spent just under five dollars on your vintage goody or more than a small fortune, you owe it to the new addition and to the rest of the wardrobe you're mixing it with to treat it with the utmost care. That means making whatever repairs are necessary, and cleaning and storing it properly to maximize the garment's lifespan. By following just a few common-sense tips and taking basic precautionary steps, you can easily bring life to a yellowed linen blouse, take years off a wrinkled cashmere coat, or freshen up a forty-year-old sweater.

REPAIRING AND CLEANING

You've just come home from a successful expedition to the flea market, your plastic bags filled with fabulous pieces you're now wondering how you ever managed to live without. You can't wait to throw on that adorable bolero jacket with velvet trim and take it out for a spin with your favorite jeans, or slip into that perfect little A-line dress with the rhinestone buttons for tonight's cocktail party. The relaxed-to-perfection khakis from a few decades back are calling out your name from the shopping bag, and that fifties tie would be perfect with the new pleated pants you just had hemmed.

Not so fast. Before you even think of leaving the house wearing any of your prized possessions, it's important to give each garment a final once-over (presumably you've already done a thorough one before you made your purchase, but it's always a good idea to double check at home, away from the thrill of the hunt). Look for small tears and holes, and whatever else you might have missed. Check for missing or loose buttons, zippers that are coming undone, and seams and hems that look iffy. Once the culprits are identified, you're much better off dealing with them right away—before you've lost a button at the restaurant or heard the seam rip as you climbed into the car. Depending of course on your sewing abilities, a button is easily secured or replaced, and a small hole quickly mended or patched. Use a small piece from a generous seam or hem, if need be. If a needle and thread are as foreign to you as the Fahrenheit conversion to Celsius, having minor repair work done is relatively inexpensive and a breeze for your local dry cleaner.

Next, check for overall cleanliness. Never, by the way, assume that a garment has been washed or dry cleaned before it was put out on the rack. With the exception of high-end consignment shops and auction houses, which tend to have more stringent demands on the condition of the items they offer for sale, it's pretty much safe to say that the last time a thrift shop or secondhand item was washed was some time before it was last worn. Check for small stains, fabric discoloration, and fading. But don't get your hopes too high. Chances are, if the garment is stained when you buy it, it's probably been stained for a while and presumably been through a few cleanings, which usually means that the stain is there to stay. But, you never know. Some stains are not forever— perhaps they were never properly treated. It's always worth a try.

Before you bring a garment into the vicinity of soap and water (or any other cleaning fluid), and before you go the dry cleaning route, look for a fabric care label inside the garment, either at the collar, waist, or on an inside seam. Be advised that fabric care instructions were not always around, so don't be surprised if you don't find one. It was in the 1960s, actually, that they made their first appearance, providing consumers with helpful guidelines for cleaning as well as fiber content information. If there's no fabric care label to be found, don't hesitate to ask the advice of someone at the store